MAN VS PROSTATE

Preserving Bladder Health for BPH

Wayne Kuang, MD

IBSN 979-8-9927244-0-0

Copy Editor Andrea Winn

Book & Graphic Design Christopher Kuang

Disclaimer

This is not a guideline. This is a community expression of support and gratitude for the expertise and experience of academicians worldwide who have paved the way for this conversation. This is an expansion of the ongoing and future dialogue among urologists, academics, and the medical device/pharmaceutical industry. This is an amalgamation of community-inspired ideas and conversations across the globe dedicated to the accelerated evolution of BPH BPO care. This is an alternate resource from which urologists can draw applicable insights for implementation within their clinical practice to better prioritize the experience for urologists, healthcare systems, patients, and their bladders.

While this Manifesto is intended for healthcare professionals, patients challenged by BPH may find this information of use. With that said, this Manifesto is not a substitute for professional medical advice, diagnosis, or treatment as it is intended for general knowledge and educational purposes only and may not be applicable to all individuals. *We recommend seeking the advice of your urologists or other qualified healthcare provider with any questions you may have regarding your medical condition. Never disregard professional medical advice or delay in seeking it because of something you have read herein.*

In the spirit of diversity, equity, and inclusion, Man vs Prostate recognizes that not all patients will identify as "male" (referred herein as "man" or "men"). This Manifesto applies to all patients with a prostate consistent with cis-male genitourinary anatomy whose bladders may be at risk for damage and dysfunction caused by BPH BPO.

The term *urologist(s)* recognizes the united effort of deobstructing urologists (MD | DO) with the invaluable supporting clinical "team" that is required to provide LUTS BPH BPO care that is personalized, effective, efficient, simple, and safe. Appreciation is expressed for "team" members that include but are not limited to the following: advanced practice providers (Nurse Practitioners, Physician's Assistants), clinical staff (Medical Assistants, Registered Nurses, Licensed Practical Nurses, urodynamic specialists), administrative staff, C-suite executives, and healthcare industry representatives and managers.

Gratitudes

Christopher Kuang An absolute joy to work with you, my son, to marvel at your skill and to see you manifest a visually pleasing experience to benefit generations of urologists and patients who suffer from BPH BPO. Unforgettable and precious. Thank you.

Andrea Winn Appreciate your time, thoughtful insights and expert edits.

LinkedIn MVP Tribe for your roles as Inspirers, Motivators, Beta Readers and Sensitivity Readers (alphabetical): Sajjad Ahmad MD, Tareq Alsaody MD FEBU, Thomas Baker, David Canes MD, Chris Carlsten MD MPH, Bilal Chughtai MD, Luca Cindolo MD PhD FEBU, Edward Cherullo MD FACS, Ed Cunha, Akhil Das MD FACS FPMRS, Hugo Davila MD, Dean Elterman MD MSc FRCSC, Carmen Gonzalez Enguita MD, Gregg Eure MD, Giovanni Ferrari MD, Steve Gange MD, Ricardo Gonzalez MD URPS, Hashim Hashim MD, Ioannis Kartalas-Goumas MD, Tommy Griffiths, Thomas Herrmann MD, Richard Hiester MA LPCC, Andrés Díaz Hung MD, Mike Jacewicz MD, Steven Kaplan MD, Mauni Keovilay, Anna Kuang MD MBA, Rob Kwasny, John Lin MD, Shawn Marhamati MD, Evangelista Martinelli MD PhD, Michael Mooreville MD, Alejandro Morales MD, Brian Murdock MBA, Helen O'Connell MD AO, Leticia Oles, Mohammed Omar MD, Sijo Parekattil MD FACS, Raj Patel MD, Joe Pazona MD, John Pfeiffer, Garrett Pohlman MD, Brad Rabin MD, David Rapp MD, Joseph Rotella MD DC, Erik Sagan MD, Milton Salazar MD, Sonny Schelin MD, Chuck Schwiesow DPT CMTPT ATC, Jason Severn, Arpeet Shah MD, Andrew Siegel MD, Jose Silva MD, Austen Slade MD MBA, Anthony Smith MD, Alexis Te MD, Peter Walter MD, Sam Warren MD, R. Charles Welliver Jr. MD, Kevin Zorn MD ... alas, I may have missed some of you...you know who you are.

By the same author

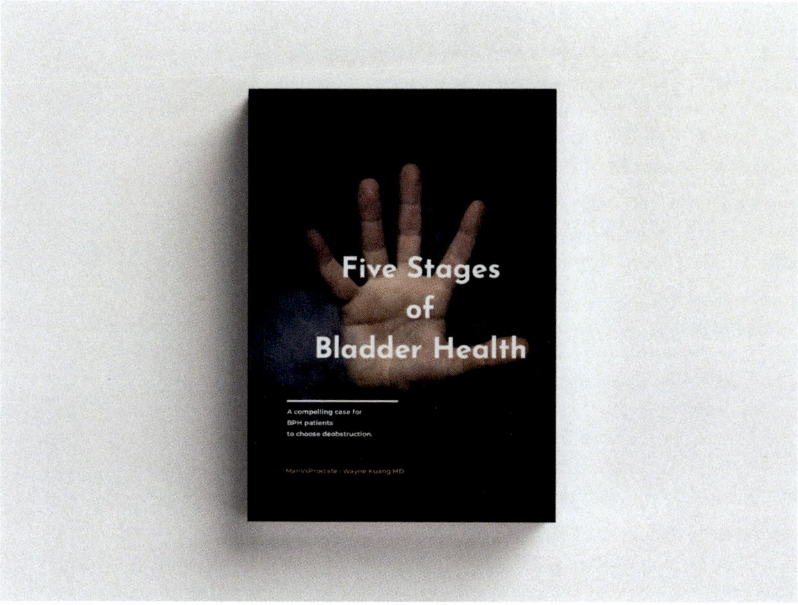

The Five Stages of Bladder Health
Free at manvsprostate.com

What readers are saying

In the MVP Manifesto, Wayne Kuang MD, brings together years of academic research, applied through a practising-urologists lens, then flips everything we thought we knew on its head. He reorients us to think more about the bladder as the critical organ to preserve, and how we should use diagnostic data to individualize care for each man sitting in front of us. As our notions of men's health evolve, we need to reconsider how we talk to and treat men suffering from LUTS due to BPO. The MVP Manifesto gives us the insight and language to do exactly that.

Dean Elterman, MD, MSc, FRCSC
Lang Family Endowed Chair in Urologic Innovation Toronto Canada
Associate Professor, Department of Surgery, University of Toronto

For me, the Manifesto is an innovative, simple and effective way to share with each patient a better knowledge of the pathological condition from which they are affected. Using the Manifesto's 5-stage bladder health histogram, I have learned to inform patients, for example in stage III, about their risk of progressing to retention or worsening of symptoms, but also about the possibility of reversing the their condition with an unblocking.... and this is true, real and extremely useful! [Translated from Italian]

Luca Cindolo, MD PhD FEBU
Consultant Urologist, Department of Urology, Villa Stuart Private Hospital, Rome, Italy
Founder, Centro Urologico Europeo, Modena, Italy

It really is time for us to save bladder function and avoid delaying surgical therapy by utilizing medications to simply cover up the problem. Just as in plumbing, a mechanical obstruction requires a mechanical intervention. With the advent of several surgical treatment options in this day and age, it is time that we step up to the plate and start to educate our patients about the need to save the detrusor.

Sijo J Parekattil, MD
Medical Director, Avant Concierge Urology, Winter Garden, USA

Man vs Prostate Manifesto is a great introduction to the complex world of lower urinary tract disorders in men. It provides awareness of the interplay between the prostate and bladder, and the complexity of management and treatment concerning it. Often overlooked is the fact that conservative medical therapy works very well and surgical options are only needed in a small minority of men. However, its identification, evaluation and treatment is paramount to preserving bladder health, and this manifesto provides a segue for patients to getting appropriate care for their prostate and bladder.

Alexis E. Te, MD
Director of The Advance Center for Benign Prostate Disease NY USA
Professor of Urology at the Icahn School of Medicine at Mount Sinai

Bladder health is an important concept that requires our attention. Many men suffer silently until they experience an episode of incontinence or urinary retention. Further research is needed to understand the optimal timing for intervention in cases of benign prostatic hyperplasia (BPH).

Bilal Chughtai, MD
Chief of Urology, Plainview Hospital of Northwell Health NY USA
Associate Professor, Zucker School of Medicine

Dr. Kuang invites readers to join an important conversation focused on the critical need for proactive and preventative care of the bladder. This dialogue serves as an important step towards progress for bladder health strategies.

David E Rapp, MD
Professor of Urology, University of Virginia Health System VA USA
Executive Director, Global Surgical Expedition

If this gets out there and gets read it is going to change the entire workup and management of BPH in a good way for urology all over the world.

Anthony Smith, MD
Former Chair, Division of Urology, Department of Surgery,
University of New Mexico
Former Chief of Urology, VA Medical Center, Albuquerque, USA

This is a very important topic. For Asian men, we suffer the same issues with neglect of our bladder health due to the fear of surgery and desire to preserve our masculinity. You have raised a very important topic.

Mohamed Omar, MD
Associate Professor of Urology, Menoufia University, Menoufia Egypt

I congratulate you on the initiative, not only for having created Man vs Prostate, but above all, for moving forward with the project by creating the Manifesto. Thank you also for having captured the way to understand this pathology simply by observing the thoughts of many of us on social media, in addition to the excellent review of the literature (Evidence-Based Medicine). The manifesto is an expression of support and gratitude towards academic urologists and healthcare professionals.
[Translated from Spanish]

Carmen González Enguita, MD
Jefe de Servicio Corporativo UROLOGIA
Hospital Universitario Fundación Jiménez Díaz (HUFJD) Madrid y
Hospitales Públicos Quirón, Salud Madrid, Spain

Author's Note

This Manifesto is the first installment of a community-inspired effort to optimize BPH BPO care to positively impact generations of men to be the best version of themselves. Through continued dialogue with patients and our peers as well as qualitative and quantitative research, this **living document** will continue to evolve.

For consistency, we use Shared Decision Making 3.0 and The Five Stages of Bladder Health throughout this document: Stage I BPO; Stage II DOA; Stage III UUI; Stage IV AUR; and Stage V DUA. Readers can benefit from first obtaining a deeper understanding by consulting the dedicated sections first.

A Note on the Author

Dr Wayne Kuang is a renowned urologist, a men's health futurist, and the founder of **Man vs Prostate**, a groundbreaking grassroots movement dedicated to revolutionizing BPH care. With a passion for preserving bladder health, Dr Kuang is committed to ending the overmedication of patients with BPH and preventing the progression to late-stage disease.

A graduate of MIT and Stanford University, Dr Kuang completed his urologic residency and fellowship training at the Cleveland Clinic in 2006. After serving as a faculty member at the University of New Mexico and a partner in a large urology group, he now cares for patients as a solo practitioner at **MD for Men**, specializing in men's wellness since 2014.

Table of Contents

Definitions 12

Our Campaign 14

Male Voiding Dysfunction 20

Prioritizing Bladder Health 28

Urodynamics 36

The Five Stages of Bladder Health 44

BPH BPO Care Pathway 56

Medications Do Not Eliminate Risk 72

Summary 76

References 78

Definitions

AUA	American Urological Association
AUR	acute urinary retention (Stage IV)
BPH	benign prostatic hyperplasia (histology)
BPE	benign prostatic enlargement
BOO	bladder outlet obstruction
BPO	benign prostatic obstruction (Stage I)
DOA	detrusor overactivity (Stage II)
DUA	detrusor underactivity (Stage V)
EAU	European Association of Urology
LUTS	lower urinary tract symptoms
mLUTS	male LUTS
PVR	post-void residual
Manifesto	a public declaration of views
MVP	Man vs Prostate®
NICE	National Institute for Health and Care Excellence

POD	post-obstructive diuresis
Qmax	maximum flow rate in mL/sec
Screening	testing of the asymptomatic to identify at-risk bladders
SDM	Shared Decision-Making 3.0
Tribe	the global group of Defenders of the Detrusor who have come together to advance the Man vs Prostate Campaign
TURP	transurethral resection of the prostate
UDS	urodynamics
UUI	urgency urinary incontinence (Stage III)
WW	watchful waiting

Our Campaign

Linguistic Determinism and BPH BPO

The Man vs Prostate Tribe respects the power of language to sculpt human choice. Linguistic Determinism highlights how written and spoken words influence how we interface with the world around us. Words shape our thoughts, which steer our clinical actions and habits. As a result, our linguistic choices can significantly shape "shared decision-making," both positively and negatively.**1** We have an obligation to carefully choose our words to uphold our *Hippocratic Oath* "To Do No Harm." In this spirit, the MVP Manifesto will henceforth explore alternate terminology as an adjunct to enhance the clinical experience for both patients and providers. Recognizing global diversity, this exploration of linguistic determinism serves as a prompt for individual countries to explore how to best use their words to honor and respect other countries' cultures and heritages to optimize patient-centered medicine.

The precedent for evolving language to shape the care for patients with BPH BPO has been cemented by urologic visionaries Drs. Paul Abrams and Alan Wein in the 1990s. In 1994, the term "prostatism" was removed and replaced with "LUTS" to recognize the multifactorial nature beyond just BPH. In parallel, the metamorphosis of "obstructive and irritative symptoms" into "voiding and storage symptoms" was witnessed.**2** In 1997, the term "the unstable bladder" transformed into "the overactive bladder" to better objectify the management for both urologists and primary-care providers.**3** Then in 1999, "a plea for the logical use of correct terms" was made to invest in properly using the terms BPH, BPE, and BPO.**4**

"BPH BPO": The histologic term BPH does not accurately convey the true nature of "BPO," which is the obstruction we urologists treat. Although the term BPO is insufficiently utilized, every

1 Li 2022; Green 2023
2 Abrams 1994
3 Wein 2011; Abrams and Wein 1997
4 Abrams 1999

effort must be made to adopt it in broader discussions to ensure precision and clarity in our communications. Although it is technically feasible to reverse the improper use of the term BPH, its entrenchment makes any attempt to resolve this impropriety highly inefficient and with diminishing returns. Therefore, it is more pragmatic to direct our efforts and resources towards tackling the main thrust of our campaign: To prioritize the preservation of bladder health for patients with BPH BPO. Henceforth, to leverage both the universal familiarity of BPH and the scientific accuracy of BPO, we propose a terminological synthesis that uses the combined term "BPH BPO".[5] Another combined term to be used henceforth is "LUTS BPH." It refers to the subset of patients with LUTS whose symptoms are suspected to be derived entirely or partially from BPH BPO. As per the International Continence Society, BPO reflects the confirmation of obstruction caused by the urethral constriction of an enlarging prostate or BPE using quantitative multichannel urodynamic testing. Later, we will similarly explore terminology such as "IPSS" and "urodynamics."[6]

Treating so much more than BPH

Benign prostatic hyperplasia is a histology term that defines the findings of proliferating glands and fibromuscular stroma at a cellular level. As urologists, our contribution to medicine is rooted in our ability to solve problems, not to manage cell types and patterns seen on a microscope slide.[7] A familiar urologic equivalent is when the kidney is blocked at the level of the ureteropelvic junction. Appropriately, it is characterized as a *ureteropelvic junction obstruction* to rationally define it by location and by the nature of the problem.[8] The use of the term *obstruction* explicitly and implicitly aligns our thoughts and actions to singularly find a solution to deobstruction.[9]

5 Abrams 1999
6 Abrams 2003
7 Abrams 1999
8 Hassen 2021; Hossain 2023
9 Foo 2017

An endopyelotomy or a pyeloplasty are performed with the primary goal of preserving renal function only after a comprehensive diagnostic evaluation is performed to have all the pertinent data before surgery (creatinine, urinalysis, CT urogram, Mag3 Lasix scan, or IV pyelogram and ultrasound). All this testing is done for an end organ that has a spare on the contralateral side and is transplantable.**10**

Another urologic correlate is a urethral stricture. Once again, a thorough evaluation is completed to collect all the relevant data that can impact surgical approach and technique (urethroscopy, retrograde urethrograms, and voiding cystourethrograms to assess location, length, and severity). The clinical presentation of urethral strictures is more acute than BPH BPO and in mostly younger men; therefore, the permanent damage and dysfunction to the bladder, the relevant end organ, is not as prevalent. While detrusor damage is rarely seen, the primary goal of intervention is to safeguard bladder health.**11** Taken together, BPO is recognized as an obstructive process similar to a ureteropelvic junction obstruction that requires a deobstructive intervention when warranted. Similar to a urethral stricture, surgery for BPH BPO is performed to preserve bladder health, which is far too often overlooked. Hence, there is an emerging global voice that recognizes the critical need to bring the oft-ignored bladder further into the spotlight. Dr Luca Cindolo in 2023 recognized the efforts of the Man vs Prostate Campaign and underscored this point in the *Journal of Nature Prostate Cancer and Prostatic Diseases* with the article "When you say 'Prostate,' don't forget to say 'Bladder!'"**12**

10 Khan 2014
11 Gelman and Furr 2020; American Urological Association 2016/2023
12 Cindolo 2023

Our Manifesto

The Manifesto is a community-inspired expression of patient-centered medicine in support of the *Guidelines of Evidence-Based Medicine.*[13] We appreciate the academic leadership for their time, experience, and expertise upon which the global guidelines have been crafted.

The precepts below are for the Guideline Committees to review and incorporate where there is merit. What was once a whisper in 2021 has received a groundswell of support and grown into a global voice to prioritize the preservation of bladder health to stem the impending worldwide surge of late-stage BPH BPO. This Manifesto aims to accelerate the transition from symptom-based to **bladder-centric guidelines.**[14] This Manifesto highlights the need to optimize the efficiency of the *pre*-treatment phase of the care pathway. This can be achieved by maximally leveraging the following measures: **screening**, **counseling**, **triaging**, and **obtaining Bladder Health Baselines**.

The Manifesto is derived from a review of the American Urological Association (AUA), European Association of Urology (EAU), and National Institute for Health and Care Excellence (NICE) Guidelines, as well as a contemporary MEDLINE search of the English-language literature. A constellation of related search terms include but are not limited to *BPH, BPO, BOO, LUTS, urodynamics, pressure-flow study, IPSS, post-void residual, uroflowmetry, screening, bladder, detrusor,* and *progression.* When multiple contrasting viewpoints are present, the Man vs Prostate Medical Advisory Committee has offered an opinion based on the most applicable and contemporary data.

13 American Urological Association 2023; European Association of Urology 2024; National Institute for Health and Clinical Excellence 2015
14 Cindolo 2023; Groves 2013; Whiting 2023

Our Vision

Patients with BPH BPO are living their best lives...chemical-free and catheter-free.

Our Mission

To *empower* patients with the educational experience:

1. To optimize bladder health and longevity with timely detection and the prevention of detrusor damage and dysfunction to preempt end-organ bladder failure.
2. To make the best decision about their prostate even faster by highlighting possible consequences of choosing not to take definitive action.

The 3 Mandates of Our Campaign

1. To preserve bladder health.
2. To prevent late-stage BPH BPO.
3. To end the polypharmacy epidemic.

Male Voiding Dysfunction

Masculinity and Decision-Making in Healthcare

Although not applicable to all men, the concept of "rugged individualism" blended with perceptions of what it is to be a man suggests that men engage in healthcare only after first donning an "armor of masculinity." BPH BPO care can benefit from a better understanding of internalized masculine beliefs that at times have been derived from the concept of men wearing this "armor."[15] Also prevalent in prostate cancer care, Chapple and Ziebland in 2022 highlighted the following masculine beliefs:[16]

1. "It was not 'macho' to seek help for health problems."
2. "The notion that 'boys don't cry' and the belief that it was not masculine to admit to weakness."

The concept of a "tipping point" has been used to describe what it takes for a male patient to engage in healthcare decisions for their medical problems. A man will endure an unnecessarily long and drawn-out period of worsening signs and symptoms for a disease process until an acute occurrence of a sudden and medically serious event occurs. This is the "tipping point." Only then will a man perceive their medical situation as dire enough to merit intervention because the symptoms are no longer acceptable or bearable. The tipping point for each man is highly personal based on past experiences, upbringing, education, and culture.[17] For patients with BPH BPO, a classic tipping point is Stage 4 Acute Urinary Retention, the sudden inability to urinate, with severe pain as urine backs up, requiring the emergent placement of a catheter into the penis and up into the bladder to drain the urine. With increased community and academic awareness of bladder health for the BPH BPO disease process, Man vs Prostate hopes that all men can avoid ever entering the late stages.

15 Le Bleu; Burns and Drentea 2023
16 Chapple and Ziebland 2002
17 Husted 2022

Balancing Patient-Centered Medicine and Evidence-Based Medicine

Evidence-based medicine has been the main catalyst for our current state-of-the-art BPH BPO global guidelines. We are grateful for the monumental effort and expertise required by academicians to implement the four-step process of evidence-based medicine:

1. Identifying a clinical problem.
2. Performing and/or reviewing high-quality research.
3. Appraising the evidence for quality and applicability.
4. Implementing clinically beneficial findings.

This approach has achieved many new diagnostic and therapeutic milestones in the recent past.**18**

Balancing evidence-based medicine with patient-centered medicine is our simultaneous focus to optimize satisfaction levels with BPH BPO care. Although a significant amount of information can be obtained digitally, in-person communication through the *Shared Decision-Making 3.0* process can clarify a patient's personal needs and wants (discussed in further detail later). These are always factored into any decision and weighted appropriately with and against other needs and wants of any other involved parties.**19**

Academic leaders have shared their concern for the lack of evidence-based research to justify alterations to reflect the importance of bladder health in the titles of global academic guidelines.**20** MVP's intention to prioritize detrusor function for patients with BPH BPO remains steadfast; however, we respect

18 Rosenberg and Donald 1995; Akobeng 2005; Sackett and Rosenberg 1995; American Urological Society
19 Brandenbarg 2020; Kalaja 2023; Hashim 2017; Wagle 2023; Abdul-Muhsin 2017
20 Ruud 2011

the academic perspective requiring high-quality proof before embracing a significant paradigm shift in thinking.

"Absence of Evidence is NOT Evidence of Absence" –Carl Sagan

With that in mind, there are instances where we must dare to take a leap of faith and implement a change, even in the absence of concrete evidence. In effect, we strive for a balance point between patient-centered medicine and evidence-based medicine.**21** We are inspired by urologist Dr Paul Abrams and his lessons learned from astrophysicist Carl Sagan. We submit the following quote for future dialogue among both community and academic urologists: "Absence of Evidence is NOT Evidence of Absence."**22** It is our fear that if we wait for all high-quality, multiyear research to come to fruition, generations of bladders will suffer needlessly, and the global consequences of late-stage BPH BPO will be insurmountable.

Male Lower Urinary Tract Symptoms (mLUTS)

The predominant pathology for mLUTS is bladder damage and dysfunction **(see Figure 1 on page 25)**. Although a detailed discussion is beyond the scope of this MVP Manifesto, it is important to recognize causative factors that can influence mLUTS directly and/or indirectly by how it first affects detrusor function. It benefits all urologists to perform comprehensive evaluations to diagnose all contributory causes of mLUTS to optimize patient care separate from or in coordination with BPH BPO care. This MVP mLUTS schematic is not all encompassing. It is submitted as a community-inspired evolutionary step forward from the landmark spoke-and-wheel LUTS schematic seen in the EAU Guidelines.**23**

21 Sacristán 2013
22 Hsu 2017; Abrams 2020
23 Harley 2018; Andersson 2011; Lee 2015; Müderrisoglu 2023;

The Aging Bladder and mLUTS

It is worthwhile to recognize the underlying progressive change seen in all bladders over time, which is simply *aging*. It is defined as "the process resulting from accumulation of consequences of life, such as molecular and cellular damage, that leads to increased risk of functional decline, chronic diseases, and ultimately mortality," and has given rise to the research field of biogerontology.**24** Although the etiologies of bladder aging include but are not limited to cellular, hormonal, genetic, and neurologic changes, recent research highlights the role of pelvic ischemia.**25** The management of mLUTS is navigated being ever mindful of end-organ changes of aging and BPO, with both contributing to symptoms either independently or in combination.

The Burden of LUTS BPH

LUTS is a widespread problem for men around the world.**26** In the Northern hemisphere, a multinational (UK, USA, Sweden) internet survey in the Northern hemisphere revealed that 47.9% to 72.3% of men (average age, 57 years) reported at least one LUTS "often" or "sometimes," respectively.**27** Meanwhile in the Southern hemisphere, countries like Brazil observed mLUTS at a rate of 69%, with 39% reporting an adverse impact on their quality of life would be "mostly dissatisfied"/"unhappy" or feel that it would be "terrible" to live the rest of their lives with the current state of their voiding.**28**

Within only a quarter century, by the year 2050, the world's population will increase by 25% from 8 billion to 10 billion.**29** The number of people over the age of 65 years will be 1 in 6 or

Messelink 2005; Hagovska 2024
24 Moqri 2023; Ranson 2015; Oh 2023
25 Kamei 2018; Suskind 2017; Nishikawa 2015; Tarcan 2022; Komninos 2014
26 Lee 2014
27 Coyne 2009
28 Soler 2017
29 United Nations

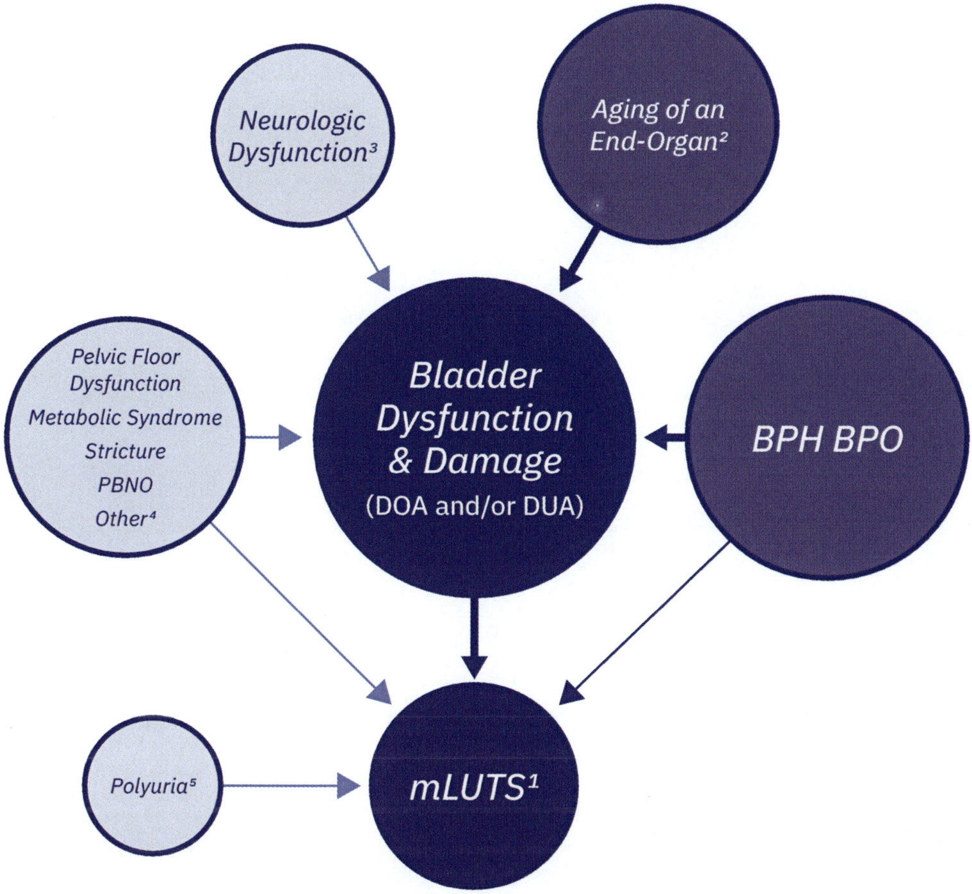

1 *Male* LUTS

2 Vascular, Neurologic, Hormonal, Cellular, etc.

3 Not Related to BPH BPO or Aging

4 Inflammatory, Stone, Dysplasia, FB, UTI, Trauma, Irritants/Allergens/Diet, CPPS, Iatrogenic, Medications, Radiation, Surgery, etc.

5 Nocturnal (OSA), Diurnal, Global

PBNO: Primary Bladder Neck Obstruction
FB: Foreign Body
UTI: Urinary Tract Infection
CPPS: Chronic Pelvic Pain Syndrome

Figure 1. Male Lower Urinary Tract Symptoms

The darkest blue circles highlight the central role of bladder damage and dysfunction in contributing to mLUTS. The darker blue circles highlight the significant contributions of BPH BPO and aging. The light blue circles underscore the multifaceted nature of mLUTS, which must be considered in all diagnostic, management, and treatment strategies.

1.6 billion.**30** With a predicted male-to-female ratio of 1:1, 800 million men will be over the age of 65 years.**31** With the global prevalence of "moderate-to-severe LUTS" being 35%, the world will be faced with the daunting task of both managing and treating an estimated 280 million of these men with significant LUTS by 2050.**32**

Global burden of moderate-to-severe LUTS in men 65 years or more: **280 million!**

Specifically, countries such as Korea, the United States, China, and the Netherlands will soon be burdened by the weight of this escalating problem as significant LUTS BPH will be seen in 25% to more than 50% of men over the age of 70 years.**33**

The worldwide impact of LUTS caused by LUTS BPH using the Global Burden of Disease database (1990-2017) estimates its burden to be almost three times more than that of prostate cancer, the disease with the next highest urological burden.**34** Another concern is the emerging data that show an elevated risk of mortality associated with LUTS. Although storage symptoms (Stage II DOA) are associated with a 1.4-fold increased risk, Stage III UUI is associated with an alarming 2.2-fold increased risk.**35**

Moreover, the global deficit of fully trained specialists is intensifying the difficulty with which we can address this surging healthcare problem. India is facing a critical shortfall of urologists. With only 5600 urologists to serve a population of 1.4 billion people, it is unsustainable to have a single

30 United Nations
31 Pew Research Center
32 Huang 2023
33 Xiong 2020; Verhamme 2002; Jeh 2024
34 Launer 2021
35 Åkerla 2022

urologist for every 255,357 persons. Extrapolating from previously mentioned statistics, there is only one urologist for every 6944 Indian men who are 65 years of age or older with moderate-to-severe LUTS. Innovative global solutions to LUTS BPH care are imperative to assist countries like India in navigating out of this predicament.**36** On the other side of the Pacific Ocean, North America is also in trouble.**37** In the United States, with its population of almost 400 million people by 2050, and assuming there are the same number of urologists then as we have now in 2023 (14,176), the ratio of a single urologist for every 783 men who are 65 years or older with moderate-to-severe LUTS is not viable.**38**

36 Singh 2024
37 Rawson 2010
38 Ortman 2009; Vespa 2018

Prioritizing Bladder Health

The Non-Transplantable Bladder

Only two major organs are *not* transplantable: the brain and the bladder. The bladder, with its intricate, afferent and efferent neural pathways, as well as its synchronized contraction and relaxation in coordination with the prostate and the pelvic floor, should be one of the most revered organs in the human body.**39** Alas, it has been unjustly ignored because the prostate continues to be the major focal point for most urologists. The time is now for us Defenders of the Detrusor to adapt, evolve, and allocate more resources to protecting the bladder, an amazingly complex and precious solitary organ.

Preempting End-Organ Bladder Failure

For centuries, mankind has aspired to "live forever". Consequently, the preservation of function for organs such as the heart, lungs, liver, and kidneys has been a top priority. As a result, many resources have been dedicated to preventing what is called end-organ failure. When this cannot be avoided, which is the worst-case scenario, modern medicine miraculously has advanced to the point of being able to transplant such vital organs.**40** Unfortunately, this is not an option for the brain and the bladder.

For obvious reasons, the vital nature of the brain has been placed on a pedestal for centuries. The bladder will never come close to attaining such a level of importance. With that said, Man vs Prostate believes the modern man wants to live not only longer, but also *better*. For patients with BPH BPO, this translates into healthy voiding that allows for a fulfilling life without the need for catheters or chemicals (medications). With a focus on patient-centered medicine, it behooves all urologists to allocate more resources to preempt the onset of end-organ bladder failure.

39 Egawa 2012; Andersson 2004; Grundy 2018
40 Mosterd 2007; Kumar 2022; Ammirati 2020

Window of Curability

Our shared prime directive is to prevent end-organ failure of the amazingly complex, solitary, non-transplantable bladder. Every patient with BPH BPO has a personalized time frame within which deobstructing therapy can prevent the onset of bladder damage or even reverse damage before it is irreparable. We call this the *Window of Curability* (see Figure 2).**41** The dialogue about the timing of deobstruction emerged in the late 1970s with classic papers by urologic leaders like Dr Paul Abrams. In 1979, he found that although prostatectomy for "prostatism" improved symptoms in 88% of patients, 25% of patients had persistent Stage II DOA and 10% had persistent Stage III UUI. It gave rise to a new avenue in thinking about whether there is a *right time* to operate.**42**

Delaying intervention beyond the Window of Curability is associated with poorer postoperative outcomes. Wasson et al in 1995 compared TURP with WW for patients with LUTS BPH with moderate symptoms in a multicenter randomized prospective trial. The TURP group demonstrated a 52% reduction in treatment failure compared with the WW group, confirming the clinical efficacy of timely deobstruction.**43** Then in 1998, Flanigan et al reported longer-term follow-up to the Wasson study and revealed insights from a crossover cohort undergoing "delayed" TURP. Similar to the Wasson study, a more than twofold increase in the failure rate was seen in the WW group (21%) compared with the immediate TURP group (10%). Of greater interest was the finding that, although the "delayed" TURPs in the WW group demonstrated clinical improvement, the degree to which they improved never caught up to those who underwent immediate deobstruction. The degree of reduction in symptom score, decrease in PVR, and gain in maximum flow rate was diminished in the crossover TURP group.**44** It suggested that there exists

41 Presicce 2017; Tubaro 2003; Bachmann and Wetterauer 2018; Stoddard 2020, Gon 2024
42 Abrams 1979
43 Wasson 1995
44 Flanigan 1998

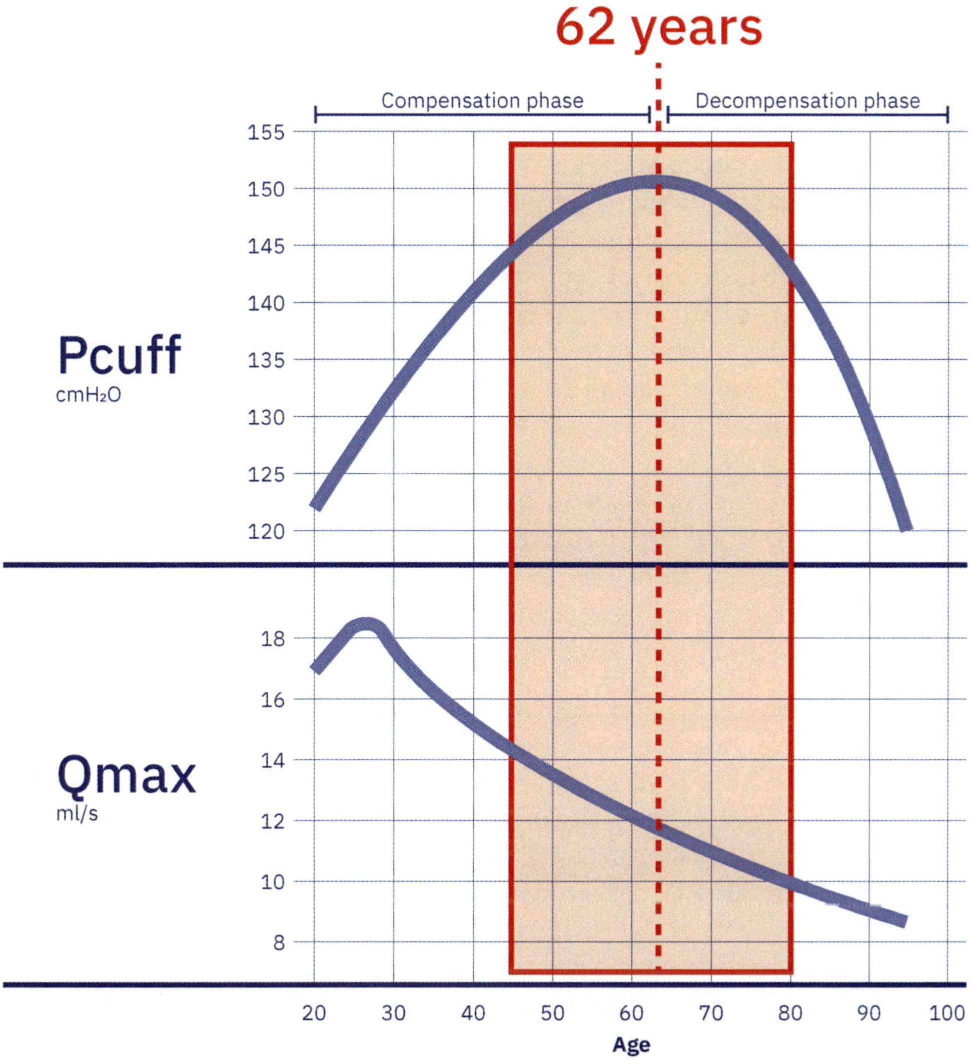

Figure 2. Window of Curability

This figure is an adaptation of the data from Kaplan 2020, illustrating the limited capacity for detrusors to compensate for bladder outlet obstruction due to BPH BPO. The x-axis represents age (in years), and the y-axis in the upper half represents isovolumetric bladder pressures (in cmH20 as measured by penile cuff test), while maximum flow rate Qmax (in mL/s) is depicted in the lower half. The blue line in the upper half depicts the compensatory rise in bladder pressures until a breaking point (at age 62) is reached, after which the decompensatory phase is entered. The blue line in the bottom half illustrates the associated consistent decrease in urinary flow rates over decades. The red box outlines a conceptual Window of Curability when applying hypothetical criteria: the earliest age at which surgery is covered is 45; and a globally accepted cut-off for an abnormal Qmax is <10 mL/sec.

a Window of Curability outside of which poorer outcomes are observed because of irreparable damage.

More recently in 2023, a retrospective cohort study by Frendl et al illustrated the negative impact of going into retention preoperatively on surgical outcomes after TURP or photoselective vaporization of the prostate. They compared 15,702 patients who had no history of catheterization preoperatively with 1772 men who had received a catheter for Stage IV AUR before surgery. The number of retention episodes was positively correlated with *treatment failure* as defined as any BPH-related reoperation or catheterization for AUR one or more months after the primary surgery. Using Fine-Gray competing-risk models, surgical failure rates at 10 years were predicted to be reduced by 31% if deobstruction occurred before any episode of AUR requiring catheterization (from 29% to 20%; $p < .001$). Timing of intervention remains a critical consideration, with a preference for deobstruction prior to any occurrence of Stage IV AUR.**45**

Landmark papers in 1991 and 1998 recognized the impact of BOO on detrusor function.**46** In 1997, Nitti et al showed post-TURP Stage II DOA could remain persistent in as much as 54% of patients, underscoring negative consequences when deobstruction is delayed for too long.**47** Thomas et al in 2005 followed patients with BOO using advanced multichannel UDS over a minimum 10-year period and highlighted the consequences when the choice is made not to intervene. Bladder dysfunction with Stage II DOA and Stage III UUI increased by 100% and 50%, respectively. Moreover, seven patients developed Stage IV AUR.**48** Inappropriately timed deobstruction often happens too late, putting patients at risk for permanent bladder damage and dysfunction, which prompted the questions of whether we are postponing deobstruction by too much and when is the optimal time to intervene.**49**

45 Frendl 2023
46 McConnell 1991; Zderic 1998
47 Nitti 1997
48 Thomas 2005
49 Gon 2024

What "Bothers" Men?

Medicine sculpted by the great minds of Hippocrates, William Osler, and Thomas Sydenham was built upon the bedrock of obtaining a detailed history as a stepping stone to an accurate diagnosis and appropriate treatment.**50** Fundamentally, history-taking was the way to ascertain what is "bothering" a patient. "*To bother*" encompasses that which causes a patient to feel annoyed, worried, or upset at something that interferes or disturbs their quality of life. Although this approach has served us well for millennia for the majority of adult and pediatric medicine, male voiding dysfunction or male LUTS has its unique challenges (as described previously) when the "armor of masculinity" results in delayed care. The tendency of men to await a serious tipping point before choosing to seek help, as well as the lack of awareness of adverse outcomes can lead to bladder damage when the choice is made to not take action on an obstructing prostate. Consequently, the use of patient-perceived "bother" as a primary outcome measure puts patients and their bladders unnecessarily at-risk. A more appropriate outcome measure centers on objecive indicators of bladder health.

Across the globe, BPH BPO academic guidelines are derived from the premise of urologists managing "bothersome symptoms." This Manifesto aims to nurture the dialogue centered around bladder health, specifically advocating for the evolution from the management of "bothersome symptoms" to the management of "bothersome fears." With the proper counseling, men "fear" five clinical scenarios:

1. The annoyance of slower flow;
2. The anxiety of urgency and frequency with the exhaustion of nocturia from an overactive bladder;
3. The embarrassment that comes with the odor and stains of urgency incontinence;

50 Ravenel 1933; Abbott and Ranson 2017

4. The terror of suddenly not being able to urinate;
5. The deep anguish of a lifetime of catheters for a non-functioning bladder.

The Stages of Bladder Remodeling

The aforementioned five clinical scenarios that encompass the bothersome fears that patients experience are often translated by urologists into academic terminology that we alone understand: BPO, DOA, UUI, AUR, and DUA. It gives us urologists the framework to discuss the pathogenesis of BPO, where BOO is a mechanical stress event. At a cellular and extracellular level, stretch-induced signals will trigger structural, morphologic, neurologic, and functional alterations via mechanotransduction pathways affecting the appearance and performance of the bladder wall.**51**

The three stages of bladder remodeling characterize the structural and functional response to BPO:**52**

Stage 1: Hypertrophic

Stage 2: Compensatory

Stage 3: Decompensatory

The natural progression through these three academic stages of bladder remodeling is unique to each patient. Fundamental to this process is the progressive deposition of extracellular matrix, including collagen as well as changes to detrusor muscle size and shape.**53** The age of onset, the signs and symptoms, the baseline bladder health, the medical comorbidities, the degree of bother, the velocity of progression, as well as the prostate shape and size are just a few of the contributing factors. Understanding each patient's personalized detrusor timeline is paramount and can be obtained with a Bladder Health Baseline for at-risk patients with LUTS. Defining the

51 Mirone 2007
52 Bosch 2018; Fusco 2018
53 Collado 2006; Blatt 2018

Window of Curability allows for preventative interventions *at the right time* to optimally maximize bladder health for our patients with BPH BPO.

These clinical data suggest a breaking point as the aforementioned compensatory stage devolves into the decompensatory stage of bladder remodeling for BPH BPO. This inflection point is around the age of 62 years.**54** More global research is needed to fill the gaps and solidify the right time to deobstruct within the Window of Curability **(see Figure 2 on page 31).**

54 Kaplan 2020

Urodynamics

Redefining "Urodynamics"

If the amazingly unique and non-transplantable bladder is permitted to have a seat at the table of Shared Decision-Making 3.0 (details to be discussed later on), the biggest challenge is allowing the bladder to "speak" and having a means to translate its needs into a "language" that allows us to take appropriate action to reconcile its problems. To do so, both patients and providers must first accept that men are not a reliable witness to their bladders. An IPSS fraught with recall bias does not accurately reflect the status of bladder health. Patients must take off their armor of masculinity and allow the bladder to give voice to its opinions through the diagnostic testing of "urodynamics." Urodynamics is the bladder's best advocate and most accurate translator.**55**

Academically, the International Continence Society defines *urodynamics* as the "measurement of all the physiological parameters relevant to the function and any dysfunction of the lower urinary tract" throughout the storage and voiding phases. The storage and voiding parts are quantitatively defined by a cystometrogram (CMG) and a pressure-flow study (PFS), respectively.**56** *Multichannel urodynamics* is classified as invasive. By default, all other diagnostics are therefore classified as noninvasive.**57**

In the spirit of Linguistic Determinism, the term *invasive* has negative connotations. The power of this word choice generates subconscious "reluctance and apprehension" for both provider and patient to pursue a diagnostic evaluation. It builds a taller wall of fear that is harder to scale to obtain necessary diagnostic testing for patients who may be at risk for late-stage BPH BPO and end-organ bladder failure.**58** Another reason to consider a supplementary definition of "urodynamics" is the dawning of the Golden Era of Bladder Diagnostics that is

55 Rutman and Blaivas 2007
56 D'Ancona 2018
57 Chung 2004; Ozawa 2010; Elterman 2013; Mahfouz 2012; Clement 2015; Whitcomb 2009; Aathi 2013
58 Cambridge Dictionary

expanding rapidly with new options. Swavely in 2019, reports 14 diagnostic technologies (seven for the voiding phase and seven more for the storage phase).[59] For Man vs Prostate, the list is one test short because it is missing one of our greatest diagnostic tools: cystoscopy. Over the last five years, the diagnostic options have continued to expand as technology becomes more advanced.[60] With so many options, it behooves us to better classify the technologies to better understand their roles in the evaluation of BPH BPO.

When BPH BPO is seen through the lens of bladder health as the centerpiece of care, even the simplest of urologic testing sheds light on the status of detrusor function, with varying degrees of precision and accuracy. With that perspective, there is a need to expand our classification beyond just "invasive" and "noninvasive." A more descriptive schema would help define diagnostic testing based on the quality and quantity of bladder data it can provide. It should reflect the range from the simplicity of IPSS to the complexity of multichannel cystometry and pressure flow studies, as well as cystoscopy.[61]

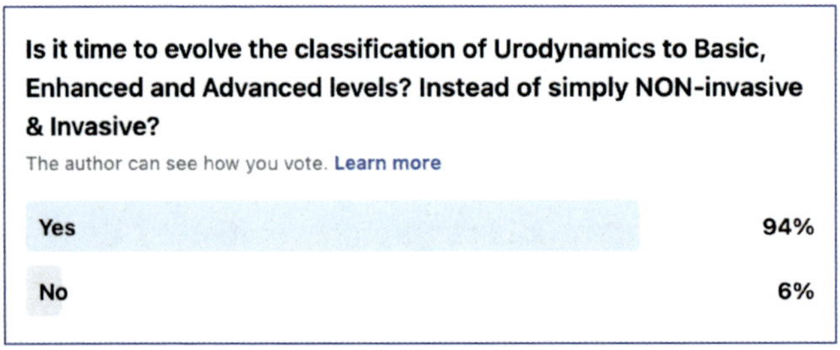

Figure 3.

In this Golden Era of BPH BPO diagnostics, a LinkedIn poll (https://shorturl.at/G4Jdx) prompted a community-based classification of "urodynamics" as defined as any test that provides qualitative and/or quantitative data about bladder health.

59 Swavely 2019
60 Frainey 2023; Kaplan 2024; Goeli 2022; Summers 2021
61 Pewowaruk 2020; Frainey 2023; Abelson 2019

The Trident of "Urodynamics" Evolving from "Invasive"

The need to evolve the classification of UDS has been proposed with a LinkedIn poll (see Figure 3).**62** From a patient-centered perspective, MVP submits this supplemental definition: "Urodynamics is any test that provides qualitative and/or quantitative data about bladder health." To reflect a progressive increase in quality and quantity of data, the classification has the three levels of "Basic," "Enhanced," and "Advanced", thus it is called the "Trident of Urodynamics".**63** Although a comprehensive discussion of all diagnostic tests is beyond the scope of this Manifesto, the most common urologic tests for the BPH BPO care pathway have been assigned to each level as follows (see Figure 4 on page 40):

1. **Basic Urodynamics**
   - IPSS, Diary, Uroflowmetry, PSA, BPHtool.com
   - 2D Imaging (PVR, PVR-Ratio, Prostate Size, Intravesical Prostatic Protrusion, Detrusor Wall Thickness, Bladder Wall Thickness)
2. **Enhanced Urodynamics**
   - CMG only: Single Channel
   - PFS only: Penile Cuff Test, External Condom Catheter and Functional Temporary Prostate Stents
3. **Advanced Urodynamics**
   - CMG and PFS: Cystoscopy and Multichannel UDS (Urethral pressure profile, leak point pressures, EMGs and video if needed)

62 Kuang, LinkedIn poll
63 Kuang, LinkedIn

Basic "Urodynamics"

Every urologist has access to some or all of the technologies of Basic UDS. These technologies assess whether a detrusor has a concerning probability of being in trouble. Basic UDS is the foundation upon which patients with LUTS can be triaged to identify at-risk bladders that need a more comprehensive Bladder Health Baseline using Enhanced and/or Advanced UDS. A detailed clinical interview and voiding diary can reveal a history of Stage III UUI and Stage IV acute urinary retention. Uroflowmetry with decreased flow rates identifies patients with Stage I BPO and/or Stage V DUA. BPHtool.com, an online

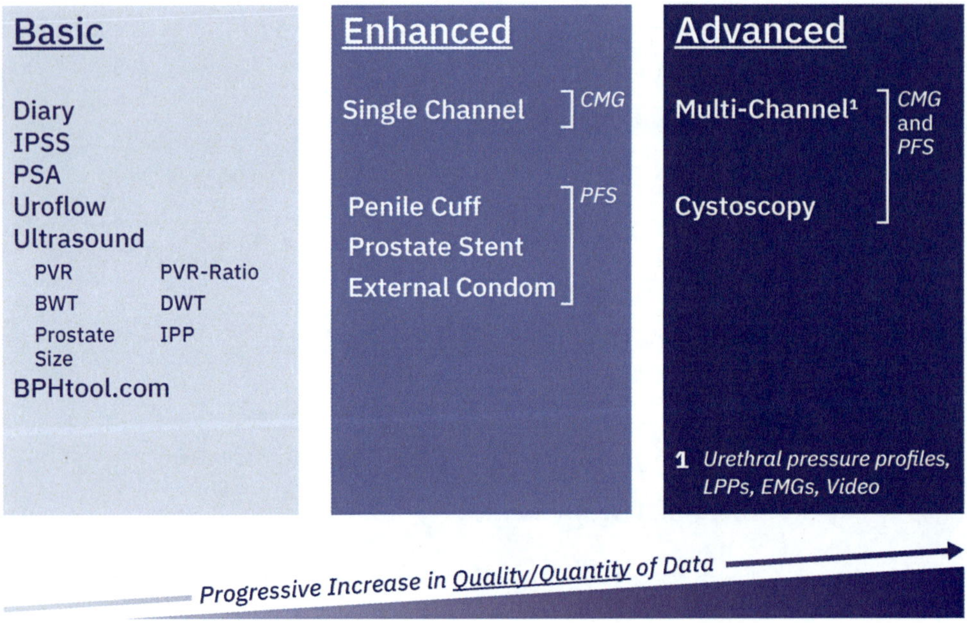

Figure 4. MVP Trident of "Urodynamics"

The Advanced level reflects data from both the filling and voiding phases of micturition. The Enhanced level is derived from either the filling or the voiding phase, but not both. The Basic level forms the core testing for bladder health screening of asymptomatic men and the Triangle of Triage to identify at-risk bladders (discussed in greater detail later on). The bottom ramp depicts the improvement of qualitative and/or quantitative data with tests above the Basic level.

tool for patients considering BPH medications, can assess the personalized risk for retention and surgery.**64**

In this dawning era of bladder diagnostics, ultrasound is asserting its leadership role within this category. Beyond the simplicity of a PVR, it is the only technology that directly visualizes the full breadth of the detrusor muscle. Every global healthcare system must develop strategies unique to their culture and medical landscape to optimally leverage these technologies for triaging symptomatic men and screening of asymptomatic men. The use of Basic UDS is a preventative measure that can minimize healthcare burden and a resource that proactively preempts late-stage BPH BPO and end-organ bladder failure.**65**

Enhanced "Urodynamics"

Beyond the "Basic" level of UDS, patients at risk for bladder damage and dysfunction can benefit from elevating diagnostics to an "Enhanced" level. Quantitative data, even if only from the voiding phase using Enhanced UDS, can be very insightful. Although it is missing data from the filling phase, a determination about BOO can be made. Two main tests are utilized: the external condom catheter method and the penile cuff test. The former has a pressure transducer connected to a condom to determine the isovolumetric pressure, a measure of bladder contractility. The latter uses a pneumatic cuff around the penis to interrupt urine flow intermittently to also determine the isovolumetric pressure. Obstruction can be visualized on a Newcastle Noninvasive Nomogram.**66** Although these two tests are unable to paint a complete picture of how the bladder functions in totality, the ability to provide data from at least the voiding phase is a definite step forward beyond the level of Basic UDS. Qualitative data about the contractile strength of the bladder are provided by temporary prostate stents. With

64 Gravas 2023
65 Bhattarai 2024; Mangera 2014; Oelke 2007, 2010; Rule 2005; Abrams 1978; Elterman 2012; Belal 2006; Malde 2016
66 Huang 2004; Mangera 2014; Pel 2002; Abrams 2004; Kohler 2023

a stent in the prostatic urethra, a successful void confirms functionally that deobstructing surgery may be warranted given that detrusor function still exists. Stents also have the added benefit of removing the morbidity of having an indwelling urethral catheter.**67**

Advanced "Urodynamics"

The highest level of qualitative data for bladder health is direct visualization with "cystoscopy." Outlet obstruction in both the heart and bladder results in muscular trabeculations. Other findings of a distressed, damaged, and likely dysfunctional detrusor are cellules and diverticula.**68**

The quantitative counterpart at the "Advanced" level is multichannel UDS. It is the most comprehensive bladder testing technology available. It can be used for all genders, all ages, and all parts of the micturition process, with an assessment of all anatomic parts including the urethra and pelvic floor. With the additional use of concomitant video imaging, it is able to provide an insightful combination of both qualitative and quantitative data.**69** It provides the highest value when performed preoperatively.**70**

67 Nguyen 2023; Schelin Cambio 2022
68 Cho 2013; Kim 2021; Ezz El Din 1996; Rahardjo 2023
69 Mahfouz 2012; Whitcomb 2009; Aathi 2013
70 Cornu 2024

Level of Diagnostics	Basic UDS	Enhanced UDS	Advanced UDS *Multi-Channel*	Advanced UDS *Cystoscopy*
High	+		+	+
Elevated	+	+		+
Standard	+			+

Figure 5. Three-Tiered Bladder Health Baseline

The Standard level of diagnostics is obtained when Basic UDS is coupled with cystoscopy. The Elevated level is reached with additional Enhanced UDS. The High level is then achieved by adding multichannel UDS. At a minimum for at-risk bladders, a Standard level of diagnostics is offered.

Urodynamics: The "Stethoscope" for Bladder Health and/or LUTS Health

Doctors in all specialties are trained to assess a diseased organ system with an evaluation of both the "structure" and "function" of that system.**71** Some blend of Basic, Enhanced, and Advanced UDS allows urologists worldwide to "listen" to the detrusor. It is a urologist's "stethoscope" for bladder health and LUTS. When patients with at-risk bladders are defaulted to the proper Bladder Health Baseline, a collective message is being established that obtaining the best available data is a paramount step in the BPH BPO care pathway.

Not every urologist and not every global healthcare system will have access to every technology within each category of UDS. With that said, cystoscopy is available to all urologists, and, as such, patients can benefit from having this test performed at all three levels of diagnostic certainty: standard, elevated, and high. These three levels correlate with the additional use of diagnostics from the categories of Basic, Enhanced and Advanced as seen with the MVP Trident of "Urodynamics (see Figure 5).

71 Woodburne 1960

The Five Stages of Bladder Health

In multiple medical specialties, classification schemes have been implemented to define the advancing severity of disease such as the American College of Cardiology/American Heart Association Four Stages of Heart Failure, the Acute-on-Chronic Liver Failure Research Consortium (ACLR-AARC) Three-Tiered Scores, The Five Stages of Chronic Kidney Disease, and the oncologic staging of prostate cancer.**72**

Similarly, the urologic literature is replete with commentary about the clinical progression of BPH BPO mirroring a linear process often seen in staging systems. In a paper by Jacobsen, Dr Claus Roehrborn in 1997 provided a visionary perspective: "I have always believed that one of the strongest motivating factors for **preventative health care** is the hope to avoid a significant, dangerous and potentially life-threatening event ... all not to correct an acute health care problem but in hopes to avoid a looming serious event in the future".**73** Moreover, in 2008, he established that "BPH is also a progressive disease, mainly characterized by a deterioration of LUTS over time, and in some patients by the occurrence of serious outcomes such as acute urinary retention and the need for BPH-related surgery".**74** BPH BPO is a progressive condition that merits a staging system to provide structure and language for communication in both the clinical examination room as well as among academic researchers. The MVP Five Stages of Bladder Health is a testament of convergent evolution, synthesizing a single unifying theme from divergent concepts: The *five* clinical scenarios that outline bothersome fears with their associated academic terminology, the *three* stages of bladder remodeling secondary to BPH BPO, and our overarching goal to preserve bladder health **(see Figure 6 on page 50)**.

To facilitate this dialogue, the description of stages *first* makes it clear that urologists unite under the common cause of preventing the occurrence of *late* stages of the disease process. Second, it then clarifies our identity not only as

72 Ammirati 2020; Hoedemaeker 2000; Kumar 2022; Mosterd 2007
73 Jacobsen 1997
74 Roehrborn 2008

deobstructing urologists but also as preventative interventionalists who intervene at the right time in the early stages of this progressive condition. Third, it communicates concisely possible adverse outcomes that can be encountered when BPH BPO is left untreated. When this is laid out on the table of Shared Decision-Making 3.0, it adds clarity to the discussion of risks and benefits in the context of possible complications, allowing for well-reasoned choices. Finally, it serves as a patient-facing educational tool that encourages men to engage sooner with a solution-finding endeavor because it outlines the consequences of inaction. Moreover, it can remove the common need for men to reach a "tipping point" in their health care before reaching out for help. The desire to avoid late-stage consequences acts as a springboard to be proactive about receiving a comprehensive diagnostic evaluation to find the correct treatment plan.

Oversimplification of a Complex Problem

For Shared Decision-Making 3.0 to be fruitful, patients must understand the risks and benefits of treatment decisions in plainspoken terms. An inherent deficiency within the process of creating a patient-facing decision-making aid is the need for oversimplification and its secondary shortcomings:

1. As seen in Figure 1, multiple factors contribute to the decline in bladder health. Although BPH BPO is a significant factor, current diagnostic technology is unable to tease out proportional contributions from other major etiologies such as the aging process of end organs, pelvic ischemia, pelvic floor dysfunction, polyuria, and metabolic syndrome. The Five Stages of Bladder Health may be overattributing undue causality of declining bladder health to BPH BPO.

2. The creation of staging systems such as The Five Stages of Bladder Health provides patients and providers a false sense of control over the overwhelming complexity of male voiding dysfunction. It is reassuring to compartmentalize

clinical consequences of BPH BPO with the illusion that every patient passes linearly from one stage to another with clear transitional boundaries. However, because of the multivariate, nonlinear, and interconnected nature of bladder function, it is duly noted that patients will likely not pass through each stage perfectly in sequence. Moreover, patients may skip over a stage, and most will present with two or more stages at one time. Patients frequently present with symptoms of both Stage I BPO and Stage II DOA. Another example is how a patient can have both Stage II DOA and Stage V DUA simultaneously, for which the term *detrusor overactivity impaired contractility* (DOIC) is applied.[75]

3. The decision to use the analogy to coronary artery obstruction (ischemic heart disease) was based on the pervasive familiarity with this disease process. Nearly every man worldwide is cognizant of the symptoms and serious consequences of a heart attack and heart failure. It is acknowledged that the more precise cardiac analogy of aortic valve stenosis could have been utilized. The benefits of a worldwide awareness of ischemic heart disease that transcends borders and cultures warrants the use of the "white lie," which is utilized for the greater good in other medical areas.[76]

4. The Five Stages of Bladder Health does not have the clarity of quantitative criteria which dictate when patients transition from one stage to another. A classic example of numerically measurable disease progression is the Tumor Nodes Metastases system used in the American Joint Committee on Cancer classification staging system. The tumor size, the number of lymph nodes and the binary presence of metastases characterize the extent and volume of the malignancy.[77] The Five Stages does not have clear quantitative threshold criteria to trigger stage escalation or de-escalation as this is only a communication tool to help patients deeply engage with their care. It does not dictate a personalized treatment plan.

75 Jeong 2021
76 Casey 2020; Nasraabadi 2024
77 Amin 2017; Hoedemaeker 2000; Singletary 2003

Advantages of Staging

Staging systems continue to play a central role in medicine by providing a language and structure to communicate both severity and urgency to clinical care. Reflecting on the benefits of oncologic staging alone, The Five Stages of Bladder Health afford multiple advantages:**78**

1. The prime directive of any simple staging system is centered around its potential to identify patients earlier, *before* the onset of bladder damage or *before* the damage is irreparable.

2. At the most basic level, a classification scheme brings order to the chaos of BPH BPO care that is rapidly growing in complexity as the number of therapeutic and diagnostic choices expands exponentially. It clearly lays out all possible consequences if the choice is made to do nothing with an obstructing prostate. It is noted that not every patient may progress through each stage, but that every patient is at risk for these clinical adverse events.

3. For many chronic illnesses, overworked primary care providers need more tools to allow for timely referrals of patients to specialists. The framework of The Five Stages of Bladder Health provides context for timely referrals with the aim of preventing the onset of late-stage BPH BPO. Specifically, an episode of UUI and/or spontaneous AUR are qualitative triggers for referral. Quantitative triggers are outlined in the MVP Triangle of Triage **(see Figure 9 on page 67)**.

4. Critical preventative strategies can preempt adverse consequences to the bladder from persistently obstructing prostates. These strategies are based on increasing awareness among the public and professionals as well as influencing policy changes and research efforts. The Five Stages of Bladder Health provides the linguistic infrastructure to support these efforts.

78 Levin 2003

5. The ability to classify a patient's clinical status based on the magnitude of the condition allows for a rationale for developing a management and treatment plan. Moreover, it systematizes research investigations with clearer metrics and improvement in clinical applicability.

6. In this era of patient empowerment, the modern man wants to take an active role in managing his own health care. The Five Stages of Bladder Health serves as an educational and clinical roadmap as patients choose to navigate their BPH BPO with the urologist as their guide.

7. Recognizing that men will often unnecessarily delay seeking help for medical care and will only do so when they have reached a "tipping point," the clinical roadmap of The Five Stages of Bladder Health serves to help men "self-ignite" sooner to seek help in an effort to avoid entering into the late stages as they recognize that their delayed choices have consequences.

8. The analogy to cardiac function and ischemic disease as described previously accelerates the adoptability and usability of The Five Stages of Bladder Health. The layperson can readily understand the similarities between the heart muscle and the bladder muscle: both act as a "pump" that moves fluid through the body—blood and urine, respectively. As stated before, a level of urgency resonates with the public when comparisons are made to a "heart attack" and "heart failure."

Stage I: Benign Prostatic Obstruction – "Things Slow Down"

Per the International Continence Society 2003 Terminology, Stage I BPO is when there is causality between the prostate and BOO. This is defined by obstructed voiding that is characterized by increased detrusor pressures in tandem with low urinary flow rates.**79** BPH BPO is a condition that progresses over decades. The prostate starts out at the size of a golf ball in the shape of a mini-donut. In the right genetic and hormonal context, the prostate grows outwardly. Of more clinical significance is when the prostate also grows inwardly, narrowing the caliber of the prostatic urethra. This can occur alone or in combination with an upward growth into the bladder classically defined as an intravesical prostatic protrusion. This makes the "donut hole" tighter, resulting in a gradual decrease in the force

79 Abrams 2003

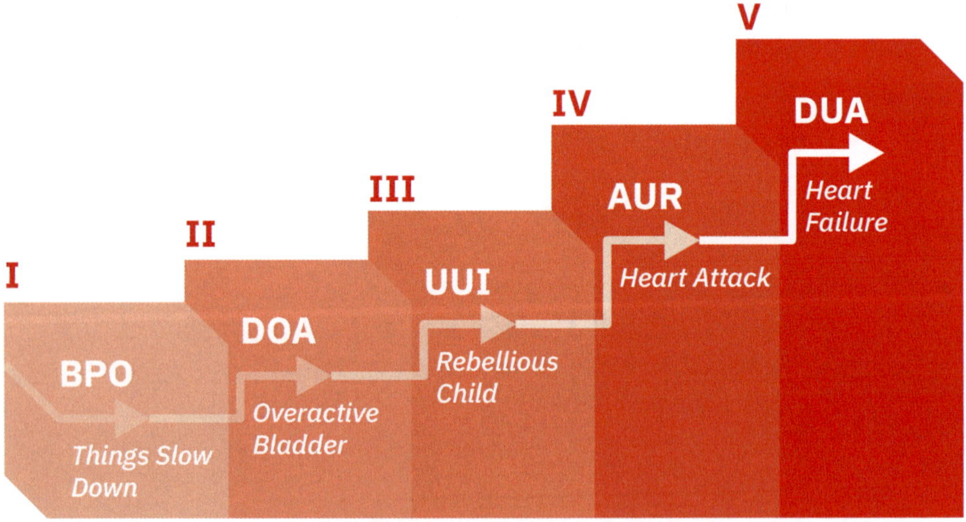

Figure 6. MVP Five Stages of Bladder Health

This patient-facing, decision-making educational aid depicts the escalation to more threatening stages of BPH BPO. It highlights possible consequences when obstructing prostates are left untreated. It illustrates the need for timely intervention within the Window of Curability. Stage transitions are not distinct, stages can co-exist, and stages can be skipped.

of urinary flow. Longitudinal studies show that as the average prostate increases in volume by 1–2 cm^3 per year, the average maximum flow rate decreases annually by 0.2 mL per second. With an increase in prostate size, "things slow down." The IPSS voiding subscore characterizes this mechanical limitation in flow with items referencing a "weak stream," "straining," "intermittency," and "incomplete emptying".**80**

Stage II: Detrusor Overactivity – "The Overactive Bladder"

Per the International Continence Society 2018 Terminology, *detrusor overactivity* is defined as involuntary detrusor contractions during the filling phase, which may be "spontaneous or provoked." The more colloquial terms *overactive bladder* or *OAB syndrome* have found a place in layman's vernacular as well as within academics to describe a constellation of urgency, daytime frequency, and/or nocturia with or without incontinence.**81** In 1991, a landmark paper titled "The pathophysiology of benign prostatic hyperplasia" foresaw a causal relationship between Stage I BPO and bladder dysfunction, including both Stage II and Stage V.**82**

Over the last three decades, research has shed more light on the generally accepted academic three resultant phases of BPH BPO: hypertrophy, a compensatory phase, and a decompensatory phase as described above that results in the Stage II DOA and Stage V DUA.**83**

Laypersons and patients can understand a "tightening donut hole" and the need for the bladder muscle to then have to generate more force to squeeze urine through a smaller-caliber opening. Over time, as the bladder muscle works harder and harder, the bladder muscle begins to struggle and "quiver" and becomes an overactive bladder. This is captured by the IPSS storage subscore with questions of "urgency," "frequency,"

80 Mochtar 20006; Gilling and Kirby 2011; McConnell 1991
81 D'Ancona 2018
82 McConnell 1991
83 Fusco 2018

and "nocturia." The prevalence of men with OAB is known to be in the range of 10% to 16%.**84**

Stage III: Urgency Urinary Incontinence – "The Rebellious Child"

Of The Five Stages of Bladder Health, this third stage deserves special attention. It can never be overstated that leaking uncontrollably on oneself diminishes a man's vitality from a physical, emotional, sexual, and social standpoint seen similarly in the experience of prostate cancer survivors.**85** Understandably, more resources are actively being allocated to the issue of incontinence in men.**86**

Per the International Continence Society in 2018, Stage III UUI describes involuntary leakage associated with "a sudden compelling desire to void."**87** This stage necessitates special attention because it has been omitted from the most globally utilized male voiding questionnaire of the IPSS. This is unfortunate because many men will never reveal this symptom unless they are prompted because of its associated shame and embarrassment. As a result, they simply continue living in the shadows with one of the most humiliating symptoms, and they accept it as part of the aging process. This is unacceptable for a symptom that has a prevalence of approximately 1 in 10 men with LUTS (11.7% in men 65-79 years of age and 18.1% for men in their 80s).**88** In 2024, the CARDIA study followed a cohort of 929 men with a mean age of 50 years and found that 3% with moderate IPSS were in Stage III UUI.**89**

Stage IV: Acute Urinary Retention – "The Heart Attack"

As per the International Continence Society in 2018, Stage IV AUR describes the sudden inability to void, often associated

84 Jaffe and Te 2006; Thomas 2005; Wein 2011
85 Chapple and Ziebland 2002
86 Gacci 2022; Kasyan 2024
87 D'Ancona 2018
88 Shamilyan 2009
89 Markland 2024

with a "painful suprapubic sensation (from a full bladder)." This is one of the most unpleasant consequences of untreated BPH BPO because there is significant pain as the result of a full bladder. Moreover, it is a burden on healthcare resources as patients frequently must rush to an emergency department for treatment.**90** Fitzpatrick et al in 2012 highlights the most common global response to retention, which is the insertion of a catheter into the tip of the penis with advancement up into the bladder to achieve relief.**91**

In the UK, the annual incidence is 3.06/1000 men, with the majority occurring spontaneously.**92** In the Netherlands, the Triumph Project revealed that the risk of Stage IV AUR was 11-fold higher for patients recently diagnosed with LUTS BPH. The incidence for this subgroup is 18.3/1000 person-years.**93** For American men with moderate-to-severe LUTS, the rates increase from 3.0/1000 person-years for men in their 40s to 34.7/1000 person-years for men in their 70s.**94**

Stage V: Detrusor Underactivity – "The Heart Failure"

As per the International Continence Society in 2018, Stage V DUA captures the scenario when detrusor pressures are low or the duration of contractions are short in association with a low urinary flow rate. The result is voiding of longer durations and/or the inability to completely empty the bladder in a normal amount of time.**95** It is estimated that the prevalence may be as high as 48% of men with non-neurogenic LUTS.**96** Patients with Stage V DUA may experience end-organ failure of the bladder caused by unnecessarily delayed deobstruction.

In this last stage, the bladder fails to perform its essential functions of storage and emptying of urine to the point that

90 D'Ancona 2018; Kaplan 2008
91 Fitzpatrick 2012
92 Cathcart 2006
93 Verhamme 2005
94 Jacobsen 1997
95 D'Ancona 2018; Miyazato 2013; Chancellor and Diokno 2015
96 Osman 2014

the patient may now be required to utilize catheters for the remainder of his life. As expected, once patients enter Stage V, they will have poorer outcomes when surgical prostate deobstruction is pursued.**97** All urologists can agree on a shared goal to not allow men to enter into this final stage, where the need for lifelong catheters would clearly not allow men to live their best lives. Moreover, it should be noted that, unlike heart failure, in which cardiac transplantation is still a last option, the failure of the bladder muscle has no such "last resort." Unfortunately, the dream of a fully functional bladder transplant that allows for "normal micturition" with coordinated control with the central and peripheral nervous system and pelvic floor is currently not on the horizon.**98**

Risk to the Brain and Kidneys

Although our staging system focuses only on the bladder, it would be remiss not to acknowledge how bladder damage and dysfunction can affect other organs such as the brain and the kidneys. Structural changes in the brain have been found in both patients with Stage II OAB and Stage III UUI. A LURN (Symptoms of Lower Urinary Tract Dysfunction Research Network) neuroimaging cross-sectional case-control study used diffusion tensor magnetic resonance imaging scans to observe microstructural abnormalities in the brain's white matter tracts within the following regions: corpus callosum, bilateral anterior thalamic radiation, and superior longitudinal fasciculus tracts, as well as the bilateral insula and parahippocampal region. It is hoped that future research will establish which interventions can reverse or halt these concerning findings in the brain.**99**

Kidneys are also at risk when bladders become damaged and dysfunctional. Late-stage BPH BPO is known to cause obstructive nephropathy resulting in Post-Obstructive Diuresis (POD). Urinary retention is the predominant presentation of POD, where polyuria is a result of a sudden decompression of

97 Chuang 2024; Thomas 2004
98 Gargollo 2021
99 Lai 2024

retention with a catheter to acutely drain the full bladder. POD is life threatening because of physiologic changes in hydration as well as electrolyte imbalances. Although the prevalence and incidence are very low, the morbidity and mortality of kidney failure are not to be trivialized, and urologists are burdened with this additional risk that patients incur when they are allowed to enter late-stage BPH BPO and end-organ bladder failure.**100**

100 Halbgewachs 2015

BPH BPO
Care Pathway

Shared Decision-Making 3.0

In all medical specialties, the choices for disease management and treatment have become challenging because of the overwhelming amount of data to be processed and the increasing number of involved parties. Traditionally, clinical decisions were made between a patient and their doctor (SDM 1.0). With the modernization of medicine, healthcare systems needed to be a part of the process to detail what resources were available and what solutions could be offered (SDM 2.0). The Man vs Prostate Campaign is predicated upon an accurate assessment for the needs of the bladder. By so doing, shared decision-making has now evolved to Version 3.0 where the bladder is allowed to take a seat at the table of clinical care because it has been established that baseline detrusor function can influence how treatment plans are sculpted and how surgical choices are made. **101, 102** A core principle for SDM 3.0 is that all parties strive for compromise attempting to satisfy as many needs as possible, but acknowledging it is impossible to meet them all.

- **Shared Decision-Making 1.0**: Patient and Urologist
- **Shared Decision-Making 2.0**: Patient, Urologist, and Healthcare System
- **Shared Decision-Making 3.0**: Patient, Urologist, Healthcare System, and Bladder

101 Brandenbarg et al 2020; Kalaja 2023; Hoving et al 2010
102 Gürbüz 2019; Thomas 2019; Malik 2019

Bladder Health Counseling

In support of our mission (stated previously), patients will need to understand the "*possible consequences of choosing to not take definitive action*" for their BPH BPO. The following basic knowledge allows patients to enter the shared decision-making process with their eyes wide open about the risk that contributes to a level of "bother" above and beyond a constellation of symptoms:**103**

1. The bladder is a **non-transplantable solitary organ** requiring a higher level of vigilance to prevent bladder damage and dysfunction.
2. BPO is a **mechanical problem** that requires a mechanical solution.
3. **Medications are temporizing measures** that do not mechanically deobstruct the prostate.
4. The **"Five Stages of Bladder Health" is a patient decision-making aid** and a communication tool to outline the possible consequences of choosing to not take definitive action about BPO.**104**
5. The shared objective for the patient and his bladder is to preserve bladder health and to **prevent late-stage BPH BPO** (Stages III, IV, or V) by intervening within the Window of Curability. This can be realized by utilizing the three drivers of good health policy: the right dialogue, the right data and the right deobstruction (see Figure 7).

103 Brandenbarg 2020
104 Cindolo 2023

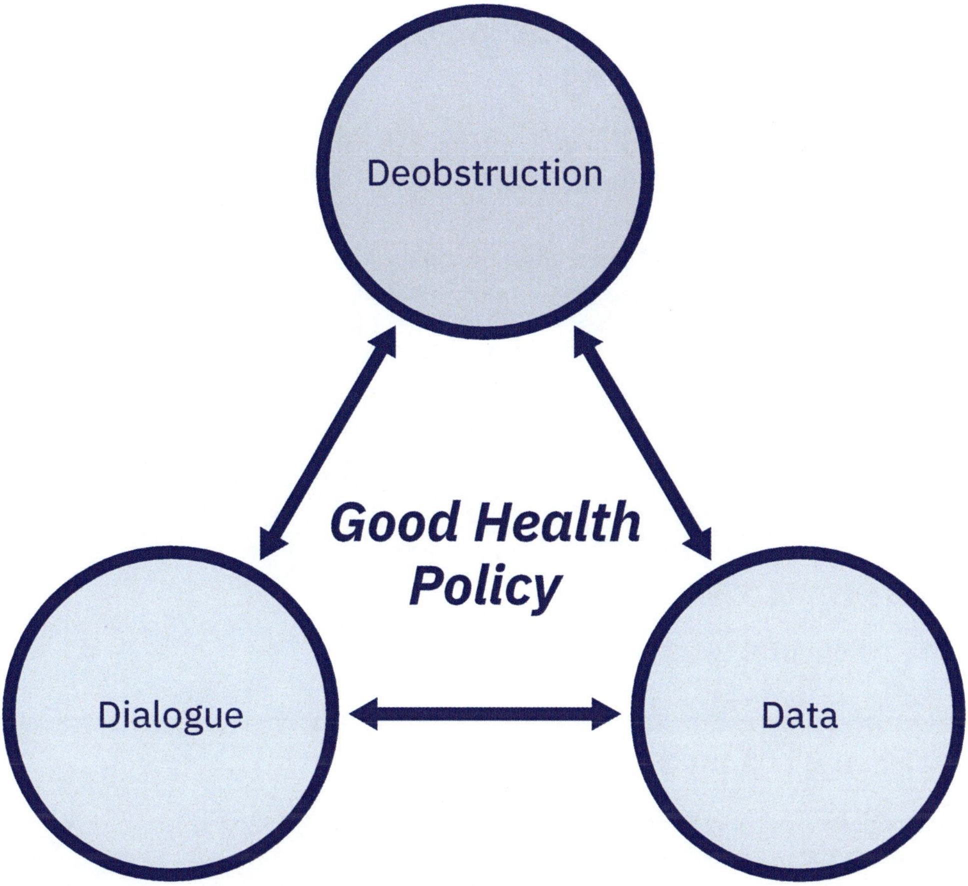

Figure 7. MVP Drivers of Good Health Policy

The pathway towards efficient and effective diagnostic management and treatment strategies for BPH BPO emerges from the convergence of the right dialogue, right data, and the right deobstruction.

The Four Elements of Good Health Policy for BPH BPO

SDM 3.0 is founded upon allowing the bladder to give voice to a patient's surgical choice. The "translation" of the bladder's needs and wants is defined by the Trident of "Urodynamics". Thus, the bladder can now be an equal partner with equal say at the table of SDM 3.0 along with the patient, the urologist, and the healthcare system.

Given the maze-like complexity of healthcare, basic precepts are needed to help guide choices with SDM 3.0. A review of the literature and all related abstracts from the AUA Annual Meeting in 2023 distilled our focus down to the "MVP Four Elements of Good Health Policy" (see Figure 8):

1. **Man's VITALITY**
2. **Treatment DURABILITY**
3. **Economic SUSTAINABILITY**
4. **Window of CURABILITY**

A man's VITALITY represents the transformation that occurs when all elements of a man's health have been optimized: physical, intellectual, emotional, spiritual, sexual, and social health. This affords men the opportunity to engage in the world with enthusiasm and vigor. For our patients with BPH BPO, a man's vitality allows him to live the best version of his life without chemicals or catheters. With this in mind, multiple studies of diagnostic and therapeutic options focus on the patient's needs and wants that must be factored into the SDM 3.0 process.[105]

Treatment DURABILITY has become an area of great interest because we have seen an explosion in the number of surgical deobstructing technologies, ranging from the least invasive to the most invasive. As we evaluate these options, we must balance risk versus efficacy. The MVP measuring stick for efficacy is

105 Rojanasarot 2023; Shore 2014; Sonksen 2015; Serati 2022

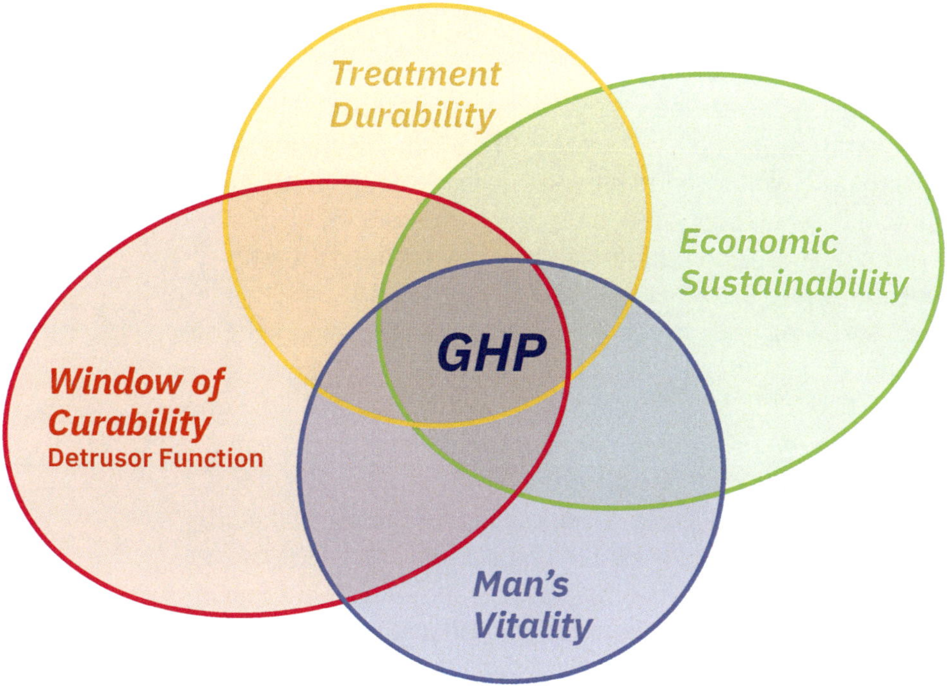

Figure 8. MVP Four Elements of Good Health Policy

This figure illustrates how good solutions are found when they are economically sustainable using durable and effective treatments. Additionally, they optimize a man's vitality when intervention takes place within the Window of Curability to optimally preserve detrusor function.

the degree to which deobstruction is achieved and how durable the treatment can last.**106** Future dialogue will need to clarify whether a second deobstruction or retreatment should be deemed a "treatment failure" if the first surgery was a product of thoughtful and collaborative shared decision-making for an organ that is known and expected to grow back via ongoing BPH.

Economic SUSTAINABILITY reflects the need for every unique healthcare system to define a BPH BPO care pathway that is cost-effective and minimizes the financial burden incurred by diagnostic and therapeutic interventions, as well as the strain felt when patients have late-stage BPH BPO and end-organ bladder failure. Of concern is how combination drugs are the

106 Kaplan 2023

least effective management strategy providing only a third of the symptom relief seen with minimally-invasive surgeries. The impact is exacerbated when BPH drugs are the most common first-line strategy, and patients are medically managed for many years without a well-defined surveillance strategy. Healthcare resource utilization analysis is a top priority as money saved for a properly managed patient can be then applied to another patient increasing the efficiency, effectiveness and sustainability of care. A growing body of research is beginning to shed light on the impact of operational changes and technological advancements for BPH BPO, often measured in quality adjusted life-years (QALYs). Although commonalities may exist, no two healthcare systems will achieve the exact same point of equilibrium given the variabilities in medical care, access to technology, and cultural differences.**107** Future research will detail whether the prevention of emergency department visits for Stage IV AUR later on in life justifies the initial cost of properly timed deobstruction earlier within the Window of Curability.

The boundaries of the Window of CURABILITY are better informed with a Bladder Health Baseline. The Baseline is defined by the Trident of "Urodynamics" and is the "stethoscope" that illuminates where a patient is within the contours of the Window of Curability. In effect, UDS is the bladder "interpreter" giving voice to whether the detrusor is weak or strong and whether it is struggling. SDM 3.0 allows for a collective choice to be made about deobstructing the right prostate for the right patient with the right technology at the right time within the Window of Curability. It should be underscored that the right time does not automatically translate to "early" since the needs of the urologist, patient, and healthcare system are also factored in.**108**

107 Cindolo 2015; Chugtai 2022; Ulchaker 2018; Wymer 2023; Wei 2005
108 Tubaro 2003; Presicce 2017; Gon 2024; Wasson 1995

Screening Starting at the Age of 50

Screening programs for chronic diseases offer many benefits: early detection with timely intervention, improved clinical outcomes, cost savings without the burden of late-stage disease, increased patient awareness and satisfaction, personalized care and health equity, optimized population health, efficiently run healthcare systems, and data collection for research.**109** In the last decade, men's health has come into sharp focus as men not only want to live longer but also better. Health screenings have evolved to include conditions such as hypertension; hyperlipidemia; diabetes; cancer (colon, prostate, skin, lung, testicle); HIV; abdominal aortic aneurysms; hypogonadism; glaucoma; and osteoporosis.**110** Understandably, public awareness through educational campaigns and social media for conditions like prostate cancer and colon cancer has been appropriately heightened given its prevalence of 1 in 8 and 1 in 23 men, respectively.**111**

Of growing concern, very few initiatives exist to elevate the standing of "bladder health," despite the alarming statistic that 1 in 3 men older than 64 years have moderate-to-severe LUTS and are at risk for bladder damage and dysfunction.**112** In 2050, this will account for 280 million men. The immense scope of this problem and the need to prevent late-stage BPH BPO and end-organ bladder failure requires effective screening measures be implemented. Man vs Prostate remains steadfast in its belief that screening guidelines should be created and implemented. Unfortunately, no such guidelines exist at this time.

As The Four Elements of optimal BPH BPO care are uniquely balanced for each healthcare ecosystem, the best age at which to start screening will require prospective high-quality research by our academic colleagues. Looking retrospectively at the

109 Miles 2004
110 Sachdev 2024
111 American Cancer Society 2024
112 Huang 2023

established literature for the incidence of Stage IV AUR based on age, screening will likely be between the ages of 45 and 55 years (global variance will exist). For simplicity and to offer a starting point, the choise to split the difference using an age of 50, which parallels many cancer screening protocols, will help ignite dialogue worldwide.**113**

Although much debate is anticipated regarding the best screening age, it behooves all community and academic urologists to agree on and unite behind a simple truth for men's health in the future: Aging men need to be screened for bladder health.**114**

Approaches to Screening

Primary care providers must be appreciated and supported for bearing the bulk of the burden of screening. Every healthcare system must find the most cost-effective means using Basic UDS tests.**115** A screening program starting at the age of 50 (range, 45-55) for each country will likely be derived from some combination of IPSS, uroflow, and PVR, with abnormal findings necessitating a urologic referral:

1. IPSS ≥8 alone *or*
2. IPSS ≥8 in combination with Qmax <15 and/or PVR >100

IPSS, Qmax, and PVR have been chosen as the primary triggers for referral given the utility of clear metrics and a lower requirement for capital. With the growth of at-home testing with hardware and/or software, audio phone apps, as well as in-office ultrasound utilization, it is anticipated that tools for screening will rapidly expand in the next decade for testing like detrusor wall thickness and bladder wall thickness.

113 Patel 2022; Kaplan 2008; Cathcart 2006; Meigs 1999;Verhamme 2005; Jacobsen 1997
114 Booth 2019
115 Triumph Trial 2024; Pell 2020

The Strengths and Weaknesses of IPSS

For generations of urologists, the IPSS has played a central role in assessing male voiding dysfunction. At this time, almost 6500 publications in PubMed cite the term "IPSS." Its greatest strengths reside in its use as an academic research tool, its ability to capture the majority of symptoms, its simplicity as a questionnaire outlined on a single side of paper, and its widespread acceptance in multiple languages among medical providers worldwide. Its limitations are rooted in the need to honor linguistic determinism and the preservation of bladder health. First, the name is inherently misleading. The International "Prostate" Symptom Score is not only about the prostate. In fact, 3 of the 7 items (43%) are about the "bladder": urgency, frequency, and nocturia.

If the name of this questionnaire were ever revised, it would behoove academicians to incorporate this precept into its renaming. Second is its inability to capture one of the most distressing signs and symptoms, which is Stage III UUI of The Five Stages of Bladder Health. Active research is determining the utility and role of ancillary questionnaires addressing incontinence like LURN (Symptoms of Lower Urinary Tract Dysfunction Research Network).**116**

Third, the IPSS is weakened by recall bias. The Greek word for recollection is "Anamnesis".**117** It captures the essence of the patient history-taking process. Alas, it is inherently flawed with "recall error" or "reporting bias" when it addresses symptoms of the bladder. Subjective symptoms remain subjective even when objectified by the IPSS. Moreover, multiple papers have confirmed the poor correlation with objective parameters gathered with the quantitative data of "urodynamic" testing.**118** Fourth, a focus on IPSS has hindered our ability to prioritize our

116 Glaser 2022
117 Wikipedia
118 Wadie 2001; Nitti 2018; Ameda 1999; Netto 1996; Fameda 1998; van Venrooij 1995

primary goal of preserving bladder health. The heavy reliance on IPSS as an academic research tool has skewed our perspective to be focused on the "management of symptoms" as reflected in all academic guidelines. As a result, much of the literature regards success as an improvement in "bothersome symptoms".**119**

Finally, the IPSS when combined with the proper counseling that includes The Five Stages of Bladder Health has the best chances of igniting patients to seek medical help for their LUTS. In Macau, China, 19-45% of men with moderate-to-severe LUTS consulted a doctor. The main reason cited for not consulting a doctor was "regarding the symptoms as normal or not problematic."**120** With the appropriate patient education including the priority to prevent the late stages of BPH BPO, men with LUTS will be empowered to take control of their health and seek the data from "urodynamics" needed to make informed choices at the table of Shared Decision-Making 3.0. In the future, the use of simplified language and/or visual schematics may improve the accuracy and precision of such questionnaires.**121**

IPSS is an Invitation

With an understanding of the strengths and weaknesses of IPSS, its true power is in its ability to prompt both patient and provider to embark on a data-first, pro-diagnostic, bladder-centric approach. It is an invitation for both to actively engage in the Shared Decision-Making 3.0 process with the healthcare system and the bladder:

1. IPSS is a perfect segue to introduce the amazingly unique, solitary, and non-transplantable organ that needs to be prioritized and taken care of. It allows for education about The Five Stages of Bladder Health, which outlines the consequences if the choice is made to do nothing about a tightening prostate. It also underscores the importance of allowing the bladder to have a voice at the table of Shared Decision-Making 3.0.

119 Cornu/EAU 2024; AUA 2023; NICE 2015
120 Lai 2011
121 Dun 2022; Park 2014

2. An IPSS ≥8 alone can be a trigger to pursue a Bladder Health Baseline with the premise that "accurate data drive appropriate decision-making."
3. IPSS covers the symptoms of Stage I BPO and Stage II DOA. It is a catalyst to inquire about a history of Stage III Urgency Incontinence and Stage IV Acute Retention.
4. IPSS allows for a natural transition in the conversation to describe the MVP Trifecta of data needed to determine possible deobstructing solutions (prostate size, prostate shape, and detrusor function).
5. IPSS is an opportunity to clearly define the role of medications as "temporizing" measures, not therapeutic measures. Moreover, it facilitates an explanation that BPO is a mechanical problem that merits a mechanical solution when warranted.

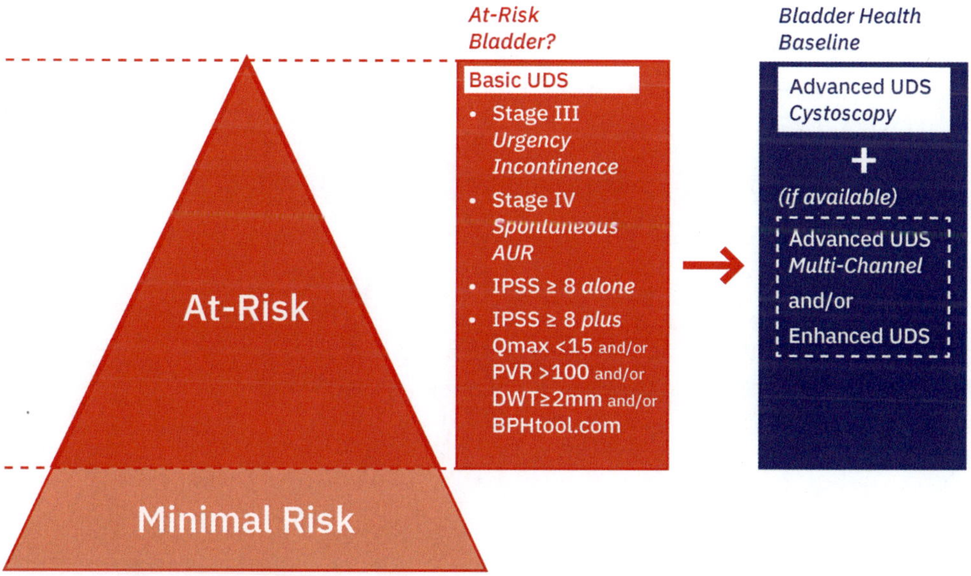

Figure 9. Triangle of Triage

Basic urodynamic metrics (red box) trigger a Bladder Health Baseline (blue box) for patients with suspected at-risk bladders (red triangle). A minimum of a cystoscopy is required for the baseline assessment. This can be elevated to an enhanced or an advanced multichannel urodynamic study, if available.

The Triangle of Triage: Identifying Bladders At Risk for Damage and Dysfunction

Screening programs provide a proactive means with which to identify asymptomatic men who may have BPH BPO. For those symptomatic men who present to the offices of primary care providers and/or urologists, the acquisition of both subjective and objective data is needed to perform a risk assessment based on the severity of bladder damage and dysfunction. This Triangle of Triage allows for timely assistance by urologists based on proper prioritization of patients and their bladders. A systematic approach allows for the efficient use of resources and efficacious care with optimized outcomes.

The Triangle of Triage aspires to incorporate the principles of high validity for risk-assessment, high interrater reliability, simplicity, efficiency of time, and a well-defined structure.**122** Any of the following at-risk features triggers a comprehensive Bladder Health Baseline evaluation that includes the minimum of cystoscopy **(see Figure 9 on page 67)**:

1. History of urgency urinary incontinence (Stage III)
2. History of spontaneous acute urinary retention (Stage IV)
3. IPSS ≥8 alone
4. IPSS ≥8 in combination with Qmax <15 mL/sec and/or PVR >100 mL and/or Detrusor Wall Thickness ≥2 mm* and/or an unacceptable risk as per BPHtool.com.

122 Ingielewicz 2024

* *Detrusor wall thickness is the representative flag bearer for other ultrasound-determined metrics such as bladder wall thickness and bladder weight that are equally viable options for specific urologists and healthcare systems. DWT anecdotally is the most commonly used in the MVP Tribe.*

A Bladder Health Baseline for At-Risk Patients

Baselines are a foundational cornerstone in healthcare. They support timely interventions to prevent consequences of late-stage disease and customize care to the individual patient. For patients who have been determined to have at-risk bladders using Basic UDS tools, a Bladder Health Baseline is indicated and includes the following Enhanced and/or Advanced UDS tools (global availability varies) **(see Figure 5 on page 42)**:

1. Cystoscopy (Advanced UDS) is an indispensable test for all levels of diagnostics for a Bladder Health Baseline and affords many advantages. First, the vast majority of urologists worldwide have access to this diagnostic technology. Second, it provides valuable qualitative data about the MVP Trifecta of surgical choice: prostate size, prostate shape, and detrusor function. Observations of protuberant "ball-valve" middle lobes, very high bladder necks, and clearly obstructing prostate lobes help accelerate the process of surgical choice. Urologists can also apply their years of experience to trust the truth of trabeculations, cellules, and diverticuli to signify a struggling bladder that is at risk. Finally, the value of diagnosing other causes of LUTS such as stones, tumors, congenital abnormalities, or strictures cannot be emphasized enough.

2. A Standard Level of Diagnostics includes the combination of Basic UDS and cystoscopy and is the minimum level of care recommended by Man vs Prostate.

3. An Elevated Level of Diagnostics can be achieved by adding Enhanced UDS tools with insights into the voiding phase (penile cuff test, external condom catheter method, temporary stents for patients with Stage IV AUR) or the filling phase (single-channel cystometry), but not both.

4. A High Level of Diagnostics can then be reached with the addition of Multichannel UDS (Advanced). This continues to be the gold standard of quantitative bladder health testing.**123** While it is always preferred given the high quality of data, it is not available to a significant proportion of urologists globally.

Urologists should aim for the highest achievable Level of Diagnostics after identifying at-risk bladders with the MVP Triangle of Triage:

1. **Standard Leve**l: Cystoscopy plus Basic Urodynamics
2. **Elevated Level**: Standard plus Enhanced Urodynamics
3. **High Level**: Standard plus Advanced Urodynamics (Multichannel)

MVP "Battle Plan"

Taken as a whole, the results of reengineering the BPH BPO care pathway to be bladder-centric can feel overly complex. To obtain clarity, a "Battle Plan" is needed to frame our approach. The Evaluation (Part One) requires proper counseling about prioritizing Bladder Health and the negative consequences when BPH BPO is left unmanaged. Symptomatic patients can be assessed for signs and symptoms of bladder damage and dysfunction using the MVP Triangle of Triage, which triggers a Bladder Health Baseline at the highest available level of diagnostics for patients at risk for late stages of this progressive disease. Subsequent Deobstruction (Part Two) is elected only when warranted after completing the process of Shared Decision-Making 3.0 while factoring in the MVP Trifecta of prostate size, prostate shape, and detrusor function **(see Figure 10)**.

123 D'Ancona 2018

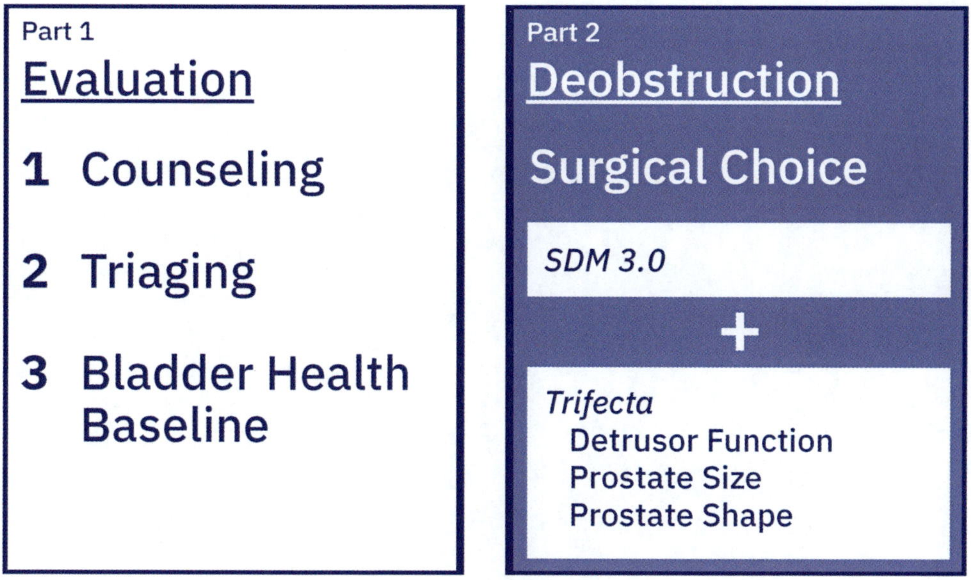

Figure 10. MVP "Battle Plan" to Preserve Bladder Health

The box on the left highlights an evaluation comprised of the correct counseling, the Triangle of Triage and the Bladder Health Baseline. The box on the right depicts surgical choice when the MVP Trifecta is factored into Shared Decision-Making 3.0 where the needs are considered for all parties: patient, urologist, healthcare system and bladder.

Medications Do Not Eliminate Risk

Modern medicine has seen the progressive increase in the perfunctory practice of prescribing, increasing doses, and refilling medications as the number of chronic diseases in our aging population rapidly increases. A consequence has been the advent of the polypharmacy epidemic seen throughout the world with rates as high as an alarming 87%. Of more concern is its association with adverse drug reactions and a decreasing benefit-to-risk profile.**124** A physician's Hippocratic Oath to "Do No Harm" highlights the true obligation to do our part in helping combat the polypharmacy epidemic by "deprescribing" when possible and finding real solutions and cures when applicable.**125**

Although other medical conditions like sepsis use drugs as a primary treating therapy (antibiotics), deobstruction is the solution that resolves the problem of BPH BPO. Bladder outlet obstruction derived from urethral-constricting prostate anatomy requires a mechanical solution when warranted. A central MVP tenet is that drugs used for BPH BPO care are "temporizing" measures, not "therapeutic" measures. Medications, similar to indwelling catheters for patients in Stage IV AUR, ameliorate symptoms and allow urologists the time to use the Triangle of Triage and to obtain a pro-diagnostic Bladder Health Baseline to fully assess the breadth and severity of BPH BPO while lessening a patient's suffering.**126** Medications are temporizing measures, not treating therapies.

This section of the Manifesto has purposely been placed at the end. This delicate adjustment relegates medications to its proper secondary position because it is not a true deobstructing therapy.

The role of medications for LUTS BPH rose to prominence in the 1990s and 2000s with pivotal studies like MTOPs and CombAT.**127** In all academic guidelines, medications play a central role in the LUTS BPH care pathway, associated with

124 Nicholson 2024; McGettigan 2024; Masnoon 2017
125 Garfinkel 2015
126 Williams 2002; Lepor 2004; Landau and Katz 2022
127 Roehrborn 2010; McConnell 2003

terms such as "medical therapy" and "first-line therapy."**128** As a result, the majority of LUTS BPH in patients is primarily managed this way. With that said, a cognitive dissonance exists in this aspect of the patient–provider relationship when only a minority of patients listen to medical advice and comply with this approach. Patients on medication for at least six months only have a one-year adherence rate of 29%.**129** This observation gives us pause, asking us to reconsider medication's role in the BPH BPO care pathway.

Within the specialty of Urology, it is popular to espouse being "minimally invasive" in our patient management styles. Although a "holistic approach" to healthcare is also often promoted, our academic guidelines prioritize the standardization of defaulting patients to a trial of drugs. MVP posits this approach is in fact "maximally invasive." This is the root of the cognitive dissonance that is pervasive in the current drug-first approach to BPH BPO care because, conceptually, these chemicals touch every cell in the body creating a plethora of adverse reactions.**130** The negative impact of medications on all systems of the human body is best exemplified by the use of chemotherapy in oncology.**131**

Although a comprehensive review of medications for LUTS BPH is beyond the scope of this Manifesto, it is worthy to note that in recent years, a growing body of research suggests the list of adverse effects to be expanding to include dementia, depression, and suicidality.**132**

Medications Sweep the Problem of BPH BPO Under the Rug

Avoidance is not a solution. For too long, medications have allowed a postponement in diagnosing and addressing the root

128 Yoosuf 2024; Singla 2016; NHS 2022
129 Cindolo 2015
130 Bortnick 2019
131 Albano 2021; Anand 2023
132 Bortnick 2019; Leibacher 2019; Laanani 2023; Kim 2020; Traish 2020; Yoosuf 2024; Mansbart 2022

cause of LUTS. It is "a wolf in sheep's clothing" to think that merely improving symptoms with chemicals will remedy a mechanical blockage or that the risk of late-stage BPH BPO will resolve on its own. One of the easiest metrics to grade the success of medications is the incidence of Stage IV AUR. In 1999, medications for patients with LUTS BPH were identified as a risk factor for retention.**133** Then over the last decade, a growing body of supporting data has shown that medications temporize symptoms or reduce the incidence of Stage IV AUR, but the risk is not eliminated entirely.**134** As a result, medications mask symptoms under the guise of "treating" a mechanical problem with chemicals, when in fact the bladder is needlessly subjected to the continuing cyclical strain due to an ever-tightening prostate.

Young et al in 2018 conducted a retrospective cohort study over two decades that showed the decreasing rate of TURP surgeries to be negatively correlated with the rise in management with pharmaceuticals. Over the 20 years, the number of TURPs decreased by 65%, whereas the number of patients taking BPH medications rose from 2% to 43%. In 1990, 65% of the TURPs were performed for the indication of earlier Stages I, II, and III, whereas in 2010, a significant shift was seen, where 68% of TURPs were performed for the late-stage indication of Stage IV AUR. Of more concern was that the number of patients who failed to void after surgery (Stage V DUA) rose sixfold from 2% to 12%. Medications when used as a "treating therapy" resulted in needlessly pushing patients to enter the late stages of BPH BPO.**135** Urologists strive to be both deobstructing surgeons as well as preventative interventionalists as we aim to uphold our Hippocratic Oath. When medications drive more patients with LUTS BPH to Stages IV and V, we must pause to consider if this is a neglect of duty to prioritize the preservation of bladder health.

133 Meigs 1999
134 Roehrborn 2010; Bauer 2021
135 Young 2018

Summary

We urologists pride ourselves in being in a constant state of forward evolution. We are experts in innovation in both action and thought. This Manifesto challenges us to rethink and re-engineer the BPH BPO care pathway in a new light as we shift away from a drug-first approach to a data-first, pro-diagnostic, bladder-centric paradigm. Our Mandates and The Five Stages of Bladder Health provide the framework to bring our patients fully into the new era of Shared Decision-Making 3.0. The Triangle of Triage and the Bladder Health Baseline allow us to "listen" to the needs of the bladder as it collaborates with us as an equal partner with equal say in shaping clinical decisions. By prioritizing the Preservation of Bladder Health, we prevent the late stages of this progressive disease and unite under the global rallying cry ... "Let's go ... Save More Bladders!"

References

Aathi MK, Devi AS, Kohli G. *Understanding of urodynamics testing.* Asian J Nurs Educ Res 2013;3(3):171-176

Abbott H, Ranson M, eds. *Clinical Examination Skills for Healthcare Professionals, ed 2.* Cumbria, UK: M&K Publishing; 2017.

Abdul-Muhsin H, Tyson M, Raghu S, Humphreys M. *The informed patient: an analysis of information seeking behavior and surgical outcomes among men with benign prostatic hyperplasia.* Am J Men Health. 2017;11(1):147-153.

Abelson B, Majerus S, Sun D, Gill BC, Versi E, Damaser MS. *Ambulatory urodynamic monitoring: state of the art and future directions.* Nat Rev Urol. 2019;16(5):291-301.

Abrams P. *New words for old: lower urinary tract symptoms for "prostatism" [letter to the editor].* BMJ April 9, 1994

Abrams P. *Good Urodynamic Practice.* May 2020. YouTube. Available at: https://www.youtube.com/watch?v=M-wY-g18R4kI&list=PL_kLLMEsNuK8SX-WaW3FVt4qO-8eT_MZ9n&index=12

Abrams P, Wein A. *The overactive bladder: from basic science to Clinical Management Consensus Conference.* Urology 1997;50(6A):117.

Abrams P. *LUTS, BPH, BPE, BPO: a plea for the logical use of correct terms.* Rev Urol 1999;1(2):65.

Abrams P, Cardozo L, Fall M, Griffiths D, Rosier P, Ulmsten U, et al. *The standardisation of terminology in lower urinary tract function: report from the Standardisation Sub-Committee of the International Continence Society.* Urology 2003;61:37-49.

Abrams PH, Dunn M, George N. *Urodynamic findings in chronic retention of urine and their relevance to results of surgery.* BMJ 1978;2:1258-1260.

Abrams PH, Farrar DJ, Turner-Warwick RT, Whiteside CG, Feneley RCL. *The results of prostatectomy: a symptomatic and urodynamic analysis of 152 patients.* J Urol 1979;121:640-642.

Åkerla J, Pesonen JS, Pöyhönen A, et al. *Lower Urinary Tract Symptoms and Mortality among Finnish Men: The Roles of Symptom Severity and Bother.* J Urol 2022;207:1285-1294.

Akobeng AK. *Principles of evidence based medicine.* Arch Dis Child 2005;90:837-840. doi: 10.1136/adc.2005.071761

Albano D, Benenati M, Bruno A, Bruno F, Calandri M, Caruso D, et al. *Imaging side efects and complications of chemotherapy and radiation therapy: a pictorial review from head to toe.* Insights Imaging 2021;12:76.

Ameda K, Sullivan MP, Bae RJ, Yalla SV. *Urodynajmic characterization of nonobstructive voiding dysfunction in symptomatic elderly men.* J Urol 1999;162:142-146.

American Cancer Society. *Key statistics for colorectal cancer.* Last revised January 29, 2024. Available at: https://www.cancer.org/cancer/types/colon-rectal-cancer/about/key-statistics.html

American Urological Association. *Urethral stricture disease: AUA guideline.* Published 2016; amended 2023).

American Urological Association. *Management of Lower Urinary Tract Symptoms Attributed to Benign Prostatic Hyperplasia: AUA Guideline.* Published 2021; amended 2023. Available at: https://www.auanet.org/guidelines-and-quality/guidelines/benign-prostatic-hyperplasia-(bph)-guideline

American Urological Society. *Clinical Practice Guideline.* Author's PDF.

Amin MB, Greene FL, Edge SB, Compton CC, Gershenwald JE, Brookland RK, et al. *The Eighth Edition AJCC Cancer Staging Manual: continuing to build a bridge from a population-based to a more "personalized" approach to cancer staging*. Ca Cance J Clin 2017;67:93-99.

Ammirati AL. *Chronic kidney disease*. Rev Assoc Med Bras 2020;66(suppl 1):S3-S9.

Andersson K-E, Arner A. *Urinary bladder contraction and relaxation: physiology and pathophysiology*. Physiol Rev 2004;84:935-986.

Andersson K-E, de Groat WC, McVary KT, Lue TF, Maggi M, Roehrborn CG, et al. *Tadalafil for the treatment of lower urinary tract symptoms secondary to benign prostatic hyperplasia: pathophysiology and mechanism(s) of action*. Neurourol Urodyn 2011 Mar;30(3):292-301.

Bachmann A, Rapoport LM, Wetterauer C. *Early surgical intervention is beneficial in avoiding complications in patients with male lower urinary tract symptoms*. Eur Urol Focus 2018;4:2-3.

Bauer SR, Walter LC, Ensrud KE, Suskind AM, Newman JC, Rickle WA, et al. *Assessment of frailty and association with progression of benign prostatic hyperplasia symptoms and serious adverse events among men using drug therapy*. JAMA Netw Open 2021;4(11):e2134427.

Belal M, Abrams P. *Noninvasive methods of diagnosing bladder outlet obstruction in men. part 1: nonurodynamic approach*. J Urol 2006;176:22-28.

Bhattarai K, Khadka H, Thapa BR, Katwal S. *Association of detrusor wall thickness (DWT) with lower urinary tract symptom severity in benign prostatic hyperplasia: a cross-sectional study*. Ann Med Surg 2024;86:3249-3254.

Blake C, Abrams P. *Noninvasive techniques for the measurement of isovolumetric bladder pressure*. J Urol 2004;171:12-19.

Blatt AH, Brammah S, Tse V, Chan L. *Transurethral prostate resection in patients with hypocontractile detrusor—what is the predictive value of ultrastructural detrusor changes?* J Urol 2012;188:2294-2299.

Booth L, Skelton DA, Hagen S, Booth J. *Identifying the most reliable and valid bladder health screening tool: a systematic review*. Disabil Rehab 2020;42:1-7.

Bortnick EM, Simma-Chiang V, Kaplan SA. *Long-term consequences of medical therapy for benign prostatic hyperplasia*. Rev Urol 2019;21(4):154-157.

Bosch R, Abrams P, Averbeck MA, Finazzi Agró E, Gammie A, Marcelissen T. *Do functional changes occur in the bladder due to bladder outlet obstruction?* ‐ ICI‐RS 2018 Neurourol Urodyn 2019;38:S56-S65.

Brandenbarg P, Rooijers P, Steffens MG, van Balken MR, Mulder H-J, Blanker MH. *What do men with lower urinary tract symptoms expect from a urologist in secondary care?* Patient Preference and Adherence 2020;14:1455-1462.

Burns SD, Drentea P. *Masculine ideals and health in older men: findings from the Wisconsin Longitudinal Study*. Am J Men Health. 2023;1-12.

Cambio AJ, Roach RM, Arnold P, Cambio J, Gluck CD, Heron SP. *Extended use of the Spanner® temporary prostatic stent in catheter-dependent men with comorbidities*. Adv Urol 2022. https://doi.org/10.1155/2022/7367851

Cambridge Dictionary. *Definition of "invasive."* Available at: https://dictionary.cambridge.org/us/dictionary/english/invasive

Casey D, Lynch U, Murphy K, Cooney A, Gannon M, Houghton C, et al. *Telling a 'good or white lie': the views of people living with dementia and their carers.* SAGE Publications. Available at: https://doi.org/10.1177/1471301219831525

Cathcart P, van der Meulen J, Armitage J, Emberton M. *Incidence of primary and recurrent acute urinary retention between 1998 and 2003 in England.* J Urol 2006;176:200-204.

Chancellor MB, Diokno A, editors. *The Underactive Bladder.* Geneva: Springer; 2016.

Chapple A, Ziebland S. *Prostate cancer: embodied experience and perceptions of masculinity.* Sociol Health Illness 2002;24(6):820-841.

Cho SY, Bae J, Yoo C, Oh SJ. *Establishment of a grading system for bladder trabeculation.* Urology 2013;81(3):P503-507.

Chuang M-S, Ou Y-C, Cheng Y-S, Wu K-Y, Wang C-T, Huang Y-C, et al. *Surgical outcomes and predictive factors in patients with detrusor underactivity undergoing bladder outlet obstruction surgery.* Int Neurourol J 2024;28(1):59-66.

Chughtai B, Rojanasarot S, Neeser K, Gultyaev D, Fu S, Bhattacharyya SK, et al. *A comprehensive analysis of clinical, quality of life, and cost-effectiveness outcomes of key treatment options for benign prostatic hyperplasia.* PLoS One 2022;17(4):e0266824.

Chung JHF, Bohnen AM, Pel JJM, Bosch JLHR, Niesing R, van Mastrigt R. *Applicability and reproducibility of condom catheter method for measuring isovolumetric bladder pressure.* Urology 2004;63(1):56-60.

Chung JHF. *Large-scale application of (the condom catheter method for) non-invasive urodynamics in a longitudinal study of changes in bladder contractility secondary to benign prostatic enlargement [thesis].* University of Rotterdam – Erasmus; 2004.

Cindolo L, Pirozzi L, Fanizza C, Romero M, Tubaro A, Autorino R, et al. *Drug adherence and clinical outcomes for patients under pharmacological therapy for lower urinary tract symptoms related to benign prostatic hyperplasia: population-based cohort study.* Eur Urol 2015;68(3):418-425.

Cindolo L, Rubilotta E, Kuang W, Antonelli A. *When you say "prostate", don't forget to say "bladder"!* Prostate Cancer and Prostatic Diseases 2023. https://doi.org/10.1038/s41391-023-00747-2

Clement KD, Burden H, Warren K, Lapitan MCM, Omar MI, Drake MJ *Invasive urodynamic studies for the management of lower urinary tract symptoms (LUTS) in men with voiding dysfunction (Review).* Cochrane Database Sys Rev 2015;4:CD011179.

Cochrane M, Drake MJ, Worthington J, Frost J, Cotterill N, Fader M, et al. *Cost-effectiveness of a primary healthcare intervention to treat male lower urinary tract symptoms: the TRIUMPH cluster randomised controlled trial.* BMJ Open 2024;14:e075704.

Collado A, Batista E, Gelabert-Más A, Corominas JM, Arañó P, Villavicencio H. *Detrusor quantitative morphometry in obstructed males and controls.* J Urol 2006;176:2722-2728.

Cornu J-N. *Preoperative urodynamics still has a role for BPH patients after the UPSTREAM trial – Pro.* French J Urol 2024; https://doi.org/doi:10.1016/j.fjurol.2024.102664

Cornu JN, Gacci M, Hashim H, Herrmann TRW, Malde S, Netsch C, et al. *EAU Guidelines on non-neurogenic male lower urinary tract symptoms (LUTS).* European Association of Urology; 2024.

Coyne KS, Sexton CC, Thompson CL, Milsom I, Irwin D, Kopp ZS, et al. BJU Int https://doi.org/10.1111/j.1464-410X.2009.08427.x

D'Ancona C, Haylen B, Oelke M, Abranches-Monteiro L, Arnold E, Goldman H, et al. *The International Continence Society (ICS) report on the terminology for adult male lower urinary tract and pelvic floor symptoms and dysfunction*. Neurourol Urodyn 2018;1-45.

Dun R-L, Mao J-M, Yu C, Zhang Q, Hu X-H, Zhu W-J, et al. Simplified *Chinese version of the international prostate symptom score and the benign prostatic hyperplasia impact index: cross-cultural adaptation, reliability, and validity for patients with benign prostatic hyperplasia*. Prostate Int 2022;162-168.

Egawa H, Tanabe K, Fukushima N, Date H, Sugitani A, Haga H. *Current Status of Organ Transplantation in Japan*. Am J Transplant 2012;12:523-530.

Elterman DS, Chughtai B, Lee R, Te AE, Kaplan SA. *Noninvasive methods to evaluate bladder obstruction in men*. IBJU 2013;39(1):4-9.

European Association of Urology. *Management of Non-neurogenic Male LUTS*. Available at: https://uroweb.org/guidelines/management-of-non-neurogenic-male-luts

Ezz El Din K, de Wildt MJAM, Rosier PFWM, Wijkstra H, DeBruyne FMJ, de la Rosette JJMCH. *The correlation between urodynamic and cystoscopic findings in elderly men with voiding complaints*. J Urol 1996;155:1018-1022.

Fitzpatrick JM, Desgrandchamps F, Adjali K, Gomez Guerra L, Hong SJ, El Khalid S, et al. *Management of acute urinary retention: a worldwide survey of 6074 men with benign prostatic hyperplasia*. BJU Int 2012;109:88-95.

Flanigan RC, Reda DJ, Wasson JH, Anderson RJ, Abdellatif M, Bruskewitz RC. *5-year outcome of surgical resection and watchful waiting for men with moderately symptomatic benign prostatic hyperplasia: a Department of Veterans Affairs cooperative study*. J Urol 1998;160:12-17.

Foo KT. *Pathophysiology of clinical benign prostatic hyperplasia*. Asian J Urol 2017;4:152e157.

Fourmarier M, Baboudjian M, Robert G, Lebdai S. *Is there a best timing for benign prostatic hyperplasia surgery?* French J Urol 2024;34:102574.

Frainey BT, Majerus SJA, Derisavifard S. *First in human subjects testing of the UroMonitor: a catheter-free wireless ambulatory bladder pressure monitor*. J Urol 2023;210:186-195.

Frendl DM, Chou WH, Chen Y-W, et al. *Early vs delayed transurethral surgery in acute urinary retention: does timing make a difference?* J Urol 2023;210:492-499.

Fusco F, Creta M, De Nunzio C, Iacovelli V, Mangiapia F, Li Marzi V, et al. *Progressive bladder remodeling due to bladder outlet obstruction: a systematic review of morphological and molecular evidences in humans*. BMC Urology 2018;18:15.

Gacci M, Sakalis VI, Karavitakis M, Cornu J-N, Gratzke C, Herrmann TRW, et al. *European Association of Urology Guidelines on Male Urinary Incontinence*. Eur Urol 2022;82(4):387-398.

Garfinkel D, Ilhan B, Bahat G. *Routine deprescribing of chronic medications to combat polypharmacy*. Ther Adv Drug Saf 2015;6(6):212-233.

Gargollo P, Butaney M, Ahmed M, Joshi V. *Feasibility study of vascularized composite urinary bladder allograft transplantation (VCA) in a cadaver model*. J Urol 2021;206:115-123.

Gelman J, Furr J. *Urethral stricture disease: evaluation of the male urethra.* J Endourol 2020;34(suppl 1):S2-S6.

Glaser AP, Kristof TW, Judge C, Javitch G, Hirsch S, Talaty P, et al. *The 10-item LURN Symptom Index (LURN SI-10) detects additional symptoms and shows convergent validity with the IPSS in men presenting with lower urinary tract symptoms.* Urology 2023;171:184-189.

Gon LM, Riccetto C. *When is the best surgical time for benign prostate hyperplasia treatment?* Asian J Androl 2024;26:119.

Goueli R, Kim MG, Goldberg K, Song C, Roehrborn C. *Real world male voiding behavior and variability using an audio-based uroflowmetry application.* J Urol 2022;207(suppl 5):e301.

Gravas S, Palacios-Moreno JM, Thompson D, Concas F, Kamola PJ, Roehrborn CG, et al. *Understanding treatment response in individual profiles of men with prostatic enlargement at risk of progression.* Eur Urol Focus 2023;9:178-187.

Gravas S, Gacci M, Gratzke C, Herrmann TRW, Karavitakis M, Kyriazis I, et al. *Summary Paper on the 2023 European Association of Urology Guidelines on the Management of Non-neurogenic Male Lower Urinary Tract Symptoms.* Eur Urol 2023;84:207-222.

Green R. *The Sapir-Whorf Hypothesis: How Languages Influences How We Express Ourselves.* August 27, 2023. Available at: https://www.verywellmind.com/the-sapir-whorf-hypothesis-7565585. Accessed May 19, 2024.

Grundy L, Caldwell A, Brierley SM. *Mechanisms underlying overactive bladder and interstitial cystitis/painful bladder syndrome.* Frontiers Neurosci 2018;12:1-11.

Gürbüz C, Drake MJ. *Where can urodynamic testing help assess male lower urinary tract symptoms?* Turk J Urol 2019;45(3):157-163.

Hagovska M, Svihra J Sr, Macko L, Breza J Jr, Svihra J Jr, Luptak J, et al. *The effect of pelvic floor muscle training in men with benign prostatic hyperplasia and overactive bladder.* World J Urol 2024;42:287. https://doi.org/10.1007/s00345-024-04974-7

Halbgewachs C, Domes T. *Postobstructive diuresis. Pay close attention to urinary retention.* Can Fam Phys 2015;61:137-142.

Harley SJD. *Identifying the predictors of change in severity of untreated lower urinary tract symptoms (LUTS) in men: a systematic review.* Paper submitted: August 2018.

Hashim MJ. *Patient-centered communication: basic skills.* Am Fam Phys 2017;95(1):29-34.

Hassen SM, Issack FH, Mummed FO, Hassen IK. *Giant hydronephrosis secondary to ureteropelvic junction obstruction, a rare occurrence, case report.* Urol Case Rep 2021;39:101803.

Hoedemaeker RF, Vis AN, van der Kwast TH. *Staging prostate cancer.* Microscopy Res Technique 2000;51:423-429.

Hossain F, Shah SS, Bastani B. *An adult case of severe asymptomatic bilateral ureteropelvic junction obstruction.* Case Rep Nephrol Volume 2023:1-3.

Hoving C, Visser A, Mullen PD, van den Borne B. *A history of patient education by health professionals in Europe and North America: from authority to shared decision making education.* Patient Educ Couns 2010. doi:10.1016/j.pec.2010.01.015

Hsu AS, Horng A, Griffiths TL, Chater N. *When absence of evidence is evidence of absence: rational inferences from absent data.* Cognitive Science 2017;41(suppl 5):1155-1167.

Huang J, Chan C-K, Yee S, Deng Y, Bai Y, Chan SC, et al. *Global burden and temporal trends of lower urinary tract symptoms: a systematic review and meta-analysis*. Prostate Cancer Prostat Dis 2023;26:421-428.

Husted M, Gray D, Golding SE, Hindley R. *reaching a tipping point: a qualitative exploration of quality of life and treatment decision-making in people living with benign prostatic hyperplasia*. Qualitat Health Res 2022;32(13):1979-1992.

Ingielewicz A, Rychlik P, Sieminski M. Drinking from the Holy Grail—does *a perfect triage system exist? And where to look for it?* J Pers Med 2024;14:590-601.

Jaffe WI, Te AE. *Overactive bladder in the male patient: Epidemiology, etiology, evaluation, and treatment*. Curr Urol Rep 2005;6:410-418.

Jacobsen SJ, Jacobson DJ, Girman CJ, Roberts RO, Rhodes T, Guess HA, et al. *Natural history of prostatism: risk factors for acute urinary retention*. J Urol 1997;158:481-487.

Jeh S, Choi M, Kang C, Kim D, Choi J, Choi S, et al. *The epidemiology of male lower urinary tract symptoms associated with benign prostatic hyperplasia: results of 20 years of Korean community care and surveys*. Investig Clin Urol 2024;65:69-76.

Jeong SJ, Lee M, Song SH, Kim H, Choo MS, Cho SY, et al. *Prevalence and urodynamic characteristics of detrusor overactivity with impaired contractility in the community-dwelling elderly with non-neurogenic lower urinary tract symptoms: is it from a single or two independent bladder dysfunctions?* Investig Clin Urol 2021;62:477-484.

Kalaja R. *Determinants of patient satisfaction with health care: a literature review*. Eur J Natural Sci Med 2023;6(1):43-54.

Kamei J, Ito H, Aizawa N, Hotta H, Kojima T, Fujita Y, et al. *Age-related changes in function and gene expression of the male and female mouse bladder*. Nature 2018;8:2089-2097.

Kaplan S, Kaufman RP Jr, Mueller T, Elterman D, Chughtai B, Rukstalis D, et al. *Retreatment rates and post-procedural complications are higher than expected after BPH surgeries: a US healthcare claims and utilization study*. Prostate Cancer Prostatic Dis 2024;27(3):485-491.

Kaplan SA, Wein AJ, Staskin DR, Roehrborn CG, Steers WD. *Urinary retention and post-void residual urine in men: separating truth from tradition*. J Urol 2008;180:47-54.

Kaplan SA, Kohler TS, Kausik SJ. *Noninvasive pressure flow studies in the evaluation of men with lower urinary tract symptoms secondary to benign prostatic hyperplasia: a review of 50,000 patients*. J Urol 2020;204:1296-1304.

Kaplan SA, Molnar GC, Shen J, Eure GR. *The role of remote diagnostics to better assess uroflow variability: insights from combining at home uroflows and frequency volume charts from 19,868 voids using a novel, hand held, cellular embedded device*. Urology 2024; in press.

Kasyan G, Grigoryan B, Pushkar D. *A novel clinical classification for male urinary incontinence: MI-CRONS*. Continence Reports 2024;10.

Khan M, et al. *Management of urete-pelvic junction obstruction in adults*. Nature Rev Urol October 2014.

Kim SJ, Kim J, Na YG, Kim KH. *Irreversible bladder remodeling induced by fibrosis*. Int Neurourol J 2021;25(suppl 1):S3-7.

Kirby RS, Gilling PJ. *Fast facts: benign prostatic hyperplasia*. Oxford, UK: Health Press Ltd.; 2011.

Kohler TS, Kausik SJ. *Comparison of IPSS score and voiding parameters in men presenting with LUTS*. Can J Urol 2023;30(5):11668-11675.

Komninos C, Mitsogiannis I. *Obstruction-induced alterations within the urinary bladder and their role in the pathophysiology of lower urinary tract symptomatology*. CUAJ 2014;8:E524-E530.

Kumar BRV, Sarin SK. *Acute-on-chronic liver failure: terminology, mechanisms and management*. Clin Mol Hepatol 2023;29:670-689.

Lai HH, Rutlin J, Smith AR, Helmuth ME, Hokanson JA, Yang CC, et al. *Structural changes in brain white matter tracts associated with overactive bladder revealed by diffusion tensor magnetic resonance imaging: findings from a symptoms of lower urinary tract dysfunction research network cross-sectional case-control study*. J Urol 2024;212:1-10.

Lai UC, Wun YT, Luo TC, Pang SM. *In a free healthcare system, why do men not consult for lower urinary tract symptoms (LUTS)?* Asia Pacific Fam Med 2011;10:1-5.

Laanani M, Weill A, Jollant F, Zureik M, Dray-Spira R. *Suicidal risk associated with fnasteride versus dutasteride among men treated for benign prostatic hyperplasia: nationwide cohort study*. Sci Rep 2023;13:5308.

Landau A, Katz D. *Prostate disease*. Healthy Male. Australian Government Department of Health; 2022.

Launer BM, McVary KT, Ricke WA, Lloyd GL. *The rising worldwide impact of benign prostatic hyperplasia*. BJU Int 2021;127(6):722-728.

Le Bleu KG. *Character, crafts, and physique: American men and the meaning of masculinity in World War I and its aftermath*. Student Theses, Papers and Projects (History). 59.

Lee H, Jeong SJ. *Epidemiology of lower urinary tract symptoms: emphasis on the status in Korea*. Korean J Urol 2014;55:300-308.

Lee JW, Kim D, Yoo S, Lee H, Lee G-H, Nam Y. *Emerging neural stimulation technologies for bladder dysfunctions*. Int Neurourol J 2015;19:3-11.

Leibacher NW, Araujo Da Silva MH. *The adverse effects of tamsulosin in men with benign prostatic hyperplasia, a review of the literature*. Am J Life Sci 2019;7(4):68-74.

Lepor H. *Evaluating men with benign prostatic hyperplasia*. Rev Urol 2004;6(suppl 1):S8-S15.

Lerner LB, Barry MJ, Das AK, Gandhi MC, Kaplan SA, Kohler TS, et al. *Management of lower urinary tract symptoms attributed to benign prostatic hyperplasia: AUA Guideline*. American Urological Association; 2023.

Levin A. *The advantage of a uniform terminology and staging system for chronic kidney disease (CKD)*. Nephrol Dial Transplant 2003;18:1446-1451.

Li J. *Relationship between language and thought: linguistic determinism, independence, or interaction*. J Contemp Educat Res 2022;6(5):32-37.

Mahfouz W, Corcos J, Campeau L. *Normal urodynamic parameters in women: Part II - Invasive urodynamics*. Int Urogynecol J 2012;23:269-277.

Malde S, Nambiar AK, Umbach R, Lam TB, Bach T, Bachmann A, et al. *Systematic review of the performance of noninvasive tests in diagnosing bladder outlet obstruction in men with lower urinary tract symptoms*. Eur Urol 2017;71(3):391-402.

Malik RD, Hess DS, Carmel ME, Lemack GE, Zimmern PE. *Prospective evaluation of urodynamic utility in a subspecialty tertiary practice*. Urology 2019;126:59-64.

Mangera A, Osman NI, Chapple CR. *Assessment of BPH/BOO.* Indian J Urol 2014;30(2):177-180.

Mansbart F, Kienberger G, Sönnichsen A, Mann E. *Efficacy and safety of adrenergic alpha-1 receptor antagonists in older adults: a systematic review and meta-analysis supporting the development of recommendations to reduce potentially inappropriate prescribing.* BMC Geriatr 2022;22:771.

Markland AD, Hellemann G, Shan L, Brady SS, Huling JD, Schreiner PJ, et al. *Characterizing the spectrum of bladder health and lower urinary tract symptoms among men: results from the CARDIA study.* Neurourol Urodyn. 2024;43(4):840-848.

Masnoon N, Shakib S, Kalisch-Ellett L, Caughey GE. *What is polypharmacy? A systematic review of definitions.* BMC Geriatrics 2017;17:230.

McConnell JD. *The pathophysiology of benign prostatic hyperplasia.* J Androl 1991;12(6):356-363.

McConnell JD, Roehrborn CG, Bautista OM, Andriole GL Jr, Dixon CM, Kusek JW, et al. *The long-term effect of doxazosin, finasteride, and combination therapy on the clinical progression of benign prostatic hyperplasia.* N Engl J Med 2003;349(25):2387-2398.

McGettigan S, Curtin D, O'Mahony D. *Adverse drug reactions in multimorbid older people exposed to polypharmacy: epidemiology and prevention.* Pharmacoepidemiology 2024;3:208-222.

McVary KT. BPH: *Epidemiology and Comorbidities.* Am J Managed Care 2006;12(5):S122-S128.

Meigs JB, Barry MJ, Giovannucci E, Rimm EB, Stampfer MJ, Kawachi I. *Incidence rates and risk factors for acute urinary retention: the health professionals followup study.* J Urol 1999;162:376-382.

Messelink B, Benson T, Berghmans B, Bø K, Corcos J, Fowler C. *Standardization of terminology of pelvic floor muscle function and dysfunction: report from the Pelvic Floor Clinical Assessment Group of the International Continence Society.* Neurourol Urodynamics 2005;24:374-380.

Miles A, Cockburn J, Smith RA, Wardle J. *A perspective from countries using organized screening programs.* Cancer 2004;101(suppl 5):1201-1213.

Mirone V, Imbimbo C, Longo N, Fusco F. *The detrusor muscle: an innocent victim of bladder outlet obstruction.* Eur Urol 2007;51(1):57-66.

Miyazato M, Yoshimura N, Chancellor MB. *The other bladder syndrome: underactive bladder.* Rev Urol 2013;15(1):11-22.

Mochtar CA. *Prognostic factors for clinical progression after treatment of BPH.* [Thesis, fully internal, Universiteit van Amsterdam].

Moqri M, Herzog C, Poganik JR, Justice J, Belsky D, Higgins-Chen H, et al. *Biomarkers of aging for the identification and evaluation of longevity interventions.* Cell. 2023;186(18):3758-3775.

Mosterd A, Hoes AW. *Clinical epidemiology of heart failure.* Heart 2007;93:1137-1146.

Müderrisoglu AE, Sakul AA, Murgas S, de la Rosette JJMCH, Michel MC. *Association of diabetes, hypertension, and their combination with basal symptoms and treatment responses in overactive bladder patients.* Front Pharmacol 2023;14:1144470. doi: 10.3389/fphar.2023.1144470

Nasrabadi AN, Joolaee S, Navab E, Esmaeili M, Khalilabad TJ, Shali M, et al. *Investigating the use of white lies during COVID-19 pandemic: a qualitative study.* Health Emerg Disasters Quart 2024;9(2):137-144.

National Health Service; Nottinghamshire Prescribing Committee. *Male Lower Urinary Tract Symptoms (LUTS) Guideline*. Reviewed May 19, 2022.

National Institute for Health and Care Excellence. *Lower urinary tract symptoms in men: management*. May 23, 2010; updated June 3, 2015. Available at: https://www.nice.org.uk/guidance/cg97

Netto NR Jr, D'Ancona CAL, Lopes de Lima M. *Correlation between the international prostatic symptom score and a pressure-flow study in the evaluation of symptomatic benign prostatic hyperplasia*. J Urol 1996;155:200-202.

Nguyen A-L, Bhojani N, Nguyen D-D, Lerner LB. *A scoping review of office-based prostatic stents: past, present, and future of true minimally invasive treatment of benign prostatic hyperplasia*. World J Urol 2023; doi.org/10.1007/s00345-023-04508-7

Nicholson K, Liu W, Fitzpatrick D, Hardacre KA, Roberts S, Salerno J, et al. *Prevalence of multimorbidity and polypharmacy among adults and older adults: a systematic review*. Lancet Healthy Longev 2024;5:e287-e296.

Nishikawa N, Yago R, Yamazaki Y, Negoro H, Suzuki M, Imamura M, et al. *Expression of parathyroid hormone/parathyroid hormone-related peptide receptor 1 in normal and diseased bladder detrusor muscles: a clinico-pathological study*. BMC Urol 2015;15:2-7.

Nitti VW, Kim Y, Combs AJ. *Voiding dysfunction following transurethral resection of the prostate: symptoms and urodynamic findings*. J Urol 1997;157:600-603.

Oelke M, Höfner K, Jonas U, de la Rosette JJ, Ubbink DT, Wijkstra H. *Diagnostic accuracy of noninvasive tests to evaluate bladder outlet obstruction in men: detrusor wall thickness, uroflowmetry, postvoid residual urine, and prostate volume*. Eur Urol 2007;52:827-835.

Oelke M. *International Consultation on Incontinence-Research Society (ICI-RS) Report on Non-Invasive Urodynamics: the need of standardization of ultrasound bladder and detrusor wall thickness measurements to quantify bladder wall hypertrophy*. Neurourol and Urodyn 2010;29:634-639.

Oh H S-W, Rutledge J, Nachun D, Pálovics R, Abiose O, Moran-Losada P, Channappa D, et al. *Organ aging signatures in the plasma proteome track health and disease*. Nature 2023;624:164-172.

Ortman JM, Guarneri CE. *United States Population Projections: 2000 to 2050*. Publication info to come.

Osman NI, Chapple CR, Abrams P, Dmochowski R, Haab F, Nitti V, et al. *Detrusor underactivity and the underactive bladder: a new clinical entity? A review of current terminology, definitions, epidemiology, aetiology, and diagnosis*. Eur Urol 2014;65:389-398.

Ozawa H, Igarashi T, Uematsu K, Watanabe T, Kumon H. *The future of urodynamics: Non-invasive ultrasound videourodynamics*. Int J Urol 2010;17:241-249.

Park YW, Lee JH. *Correlation between the Visual Prostate Symptom Score and International Prostate Symptom Score in patients with lower urinary tract symptoms*. Int Neurourol J 2014;18(1):37-41.

Patel AV, Deubler E, Teras LR, Colditz GA, Lichtman CJ, Cance WG, et al. *Key risk factors for the relative and absolute 5-year risk of cancer to enhance cancer screening and prevention*. Cancer 2022;128(19):3502-3515

Pel JJM, Bosch JLHR, Blom JHM, Lycklama à Nijeholt AAB, van Mastrigt R. *Development of a non-invasive strategy to classify bladder outlet obstruction in male patients with LUTS*. Neurourol Urodyn 2022;21(2):117-125.

Pell B, Thomas-Jones E, Bray A, Agarwal R, Ahmed H, Allen AJ, et al. *PRImary care Management of lower Urinary tract Symptoms in men: protocol for development and validation of a diagnostic and clinical decision support tool (the PriMUS study)*. BMJ Open 2020;10:e037634.

Pew Research Center. *Global population skews male, but UN projects parity between sexes by 2050*. Available at: https://www.pewresearch.org/short-reads/2022/08/31/global-population-skews-male-but-un-projects-parity-between-sexes-by-2050/#:~:text=But%20by%202050%2C%20the%20worldwide,females%20in%20the%20global%20population

Pewowaruk R, Rutkowski D, Hernando D, Kumapayi BB, Bushman W, Roldán-Alzate A. *A pilot study of bladder voiding with real-time MRI and computational fluid dynamics*. PLoS One 2020;15(11):e0238404.

Presicce F, De Nunzio C, Gacci M, Sosnowsky R, Lombardo R, Porpiglia F, et al. *The influence of the medical treatment of LUTS on benign prostatic hyperplasia surgery: do we operate too late?* Minerva Urologica e Nefrologica 2017;69(3):242-252.

Rahardjo HE, Märker V, Tsikas D, Kuczyk MA, Ückert S, Bannowsky A. *Fibrotic diseases of the human urinary and genital tract: current understanding and potential strategies for treatment*. J Clin Med 2023;12:4770.

Ranson RN, Saffrey MJ. *Neurogenic mechanisms in bladder and bowel ageing*. Biogerontology 2015;16:265-284.

Ravenel MP. Review. Sigerist HE. *The Great Doctors. A Biographical History of Medicine*. New York: Norton; 1933. 436 pp.

Rawson NSB, Saad F. *The aging male population and medical care for benign prostatic hyperplasia in Canada*. Can Urol Assoc J 2010;4(2):123-127.

Roehrborn CG. *BPH progression: concept and key learning from MTOPS, ALTESS, COMBAT, and ALF-ONE*. BJU Int 2008;101(suppl 3):17-21.

Roehrborn CG, Siami P, Barkin J, Damião R, Major-Walker K, Nandy I, et al. *The effects of combination therapy with dutasteride and tamsulosin on clinical outcomes in men with symptomatic benign prostatic hyperplasia: 4-year results from the CombAT Study*. Eur Urol 2010;57(1):123-131.

Rojanasarot S, Cutone B, Durand K, Zorn KC, Chughtai B, Bhojani N, et al. *Patients' perspectives on attributes while choosing minimally invasive surgery for benign prostatic hyperplasia procedures: experience from men undergoing water vapor thermal therapy*. J Endourol 2023;3l7(5):575-580.

Rosenberg W, Donald A. *Evidence based medicine: an approach to clinical problem-solving*. BMJ 1995;310(1):122-126.

Rule AD, Jacobson DJ, McGree ME, Girman CJ, Lieber MM, Jacobsen SJ. *Longitudinal changes in post-void residual and voided volume among community dwelling men*. J Urol 2005;174:1317-1322.

Rutman MP, Blaivas JG. *Urodynamics: what to do and when is it clinically necessary?* Curr Urol Rep 2007;8:263-268.

Ruud Bosch JLH, Cardozo L, Hashim H, Hilton P, Oelke M, Robinson D. *Constructing trials to show whether urodynamic studies are necessary in lower urinary tract dysfunction*. Neurourol Urodynamics 2011;30:735-740.

Sachdev P. *Slideshow: Essential Screening Tests Every Man Needs*. WebMD. March 10, 2024. Available at: https://www.webmd.com/men/ss/slideshow-screening-tests-men

Sackett DL, Rosenberg WMC. *The need for evidence-based medicine*. J R Soc Med 1995;88:620-624.

Sacristán JA. *Medicina basada en la evidencia y medicina centrada en el paciente: algunas reflexiones sobre su integración*. Rev Clin Esp 2013;213:460-464.

Schelin S. *CoreFlow Soft Stent® used as a persistent catheter substitute for 11 months waiting for surgery: spontaneous micturition and full continence without UTI resulted*. Mega Journal of Case Reports 2023.

Serati M, Braga A, Rosier PFWM, de Wachter S, Uren A, FinazziAgrò E. *Acceptability and perceived value of urodynamics from the patient perspective: a narrative review*. Neurourol Urodyn 2022; DOI: 10.1002/nau.24932.

Shamliyan TA, Wyman JF, Ping R, Wilt TJ, Kane RL. *Male urinary incontinence: prevalence, risk factors, and preventive interventions*. Rev Urol 2009;11(3):145-165.

Shore N, Freedman S, Gange S, Moseley W, Heron S, Tutrone R, et al. *Prospective multi-center study elucidating patient experience after prostatic urethral lift*. Can J Urol 2014;21(1):7094-7101.

Singh S. *Urology around the world: India: past, present, and future*. Urology News. January 23, 2024. Available at: https://www.urologynews.uk.com/features/features/post/urology-around-the-world-india-past-present-and-future

Singla N, Singla AK. *Evaluation and management of lower urinary tract symptoms after outlet surgery for benign prostatic hyperplasia*. Curr Bladder Dysfunct Rep 2016;11(3):242-247.

Singletary SE, Allred C, Ashley P, Bassett LW, Berry D, Bland KI, et al. *Staging system for breast cancer: revisions for the 6th edition of the AJCC Cancer Staging Manual*. Surg Clin N Am 2003;83:803-819.

Soler R, Mendes Gomes C, Averbeck MA, Koyama M. *The prevalence of lower urinary tract symptoms (LUTS) in Brazil: results from the epidemiology of LUTS (Brazil LUTS) study*. Neurourol Urodyn. 2018;37:1356-1364.

Sønksen J, Barber NJ, Speakman MJ, Berges R, Wetterauer U, Greene D, et al. *Prospective, randomized, multinational study of prostatic urethral lift versus transurethral resection of the prostate: 12-month results from the BPH6 study*. Eur Urol 2015;68:643-652.

Stoddard MD, Cho A, Te AE, Chughtai B. *A systematic review on the timing of surgical intervention for benign prostatic enlargement (BPE)*. Curr Urol Rep 2020;21:64.

Summers SJ, Armstrong JM, Kaplan SA, Te AE, Le A, Heiner SM, et al. *Male voiding behavior: insight from 19,824 at-home Uroflow profiles*. J Urol 2021;205:1126-1132.

Suskind AM. *The aging overactive bladder: a review of aging-related changes from the brain to the bladder*. Curr Bladder Dysfunction Rep 2017;12:42-47.

Swavely NR, Speich JE, Stothers L, Klausner AP. *New diagnostics for male lower urinary tract symptoms*. Curr Bladder Dysfunct Rep 2019;14:90-97.

Tarcan T, Choi H-P, Azadzoi KM. *Molecular regulation of concomitant lower urinary tract symptoms and erectile dysfunction in pelvic ischemia*. Int J Mol Sci 2022;23:15988.

Thomas AW, Cannon A, Bartlett E, Ellis-Jones J, Abrams P. *The natural history of lower urinary tract dysfunction in men: minimum 10-year urodynamic follow-up of untreated bladder outlet obstruction*. BJU Int 2005;96:1301-1306.

Thomas D, Zorn KC, Zaidi N, Chen SA, Zhang Y, Te A, et al. *Does urodynamics predict voiding after benign prostatic hyperplasia surgery in patients with detrusor underactivity?* Asian J Urol 2019;6:264-269.

Traish AM. *Post-finasteride syndrome: a surmountable challenge for clinicians*. Fertil Steril 2020;113(1):21-50.

Tubaro A, Carter S, Trucchi A, Punzo G, Petta S, Miano L. *Early treatment of benign prostatic hyperplasia. Implications for reducing the risk of permanent bladder damage*. Drugs Aging 2003;20(3):185-195.

Ulchaker JC, Martinson MS. *Cost-effectiveness analysis of six therapies for the treatment of lower urinary tract symptoms due to benign prostatic hyperplasia*. Clinicoecon Outcomes Res. 2018;10:29-43 https://doi.org/10.2147/CEOR.S148195

United Nations. *Global Issues*. Population. Available at: https://www.un.org/en/global-issues/population#:~:text=The%20world's%20population%20is%20expected,billion%20in%20the%20mid%2D2080s

United Nations. *Our world is growing older: UN DESA releases new report on ageing*. Available at: https://www.un.org/development/desa/en/news/population/our-world-is-growing-older.html#:~:text=Today%2C%20there%20are%20703%20million,1%20in%2011%20in%202019

van Venrooij GEPM, Boon TA, de Gier RPE. *International Prostate Symptom Score and quality of life assessment versus urodynamic parameters in men with benign prostatic hyperplasia symptoms*. J Urol 1995;153:1516-1519.

Verhamme KMC, Dieleman JP, Bleumink GS, van der Lei J, Sturkenboom MCJM; *Triumph Pan European Expert Panel*. Eur Urol 2002;42(4):323-328.

Verhamme KMC, Dieleman JP, van Wijk MAM, Bosch JLHR, Stricker BHCh, Sturkenboom MCJM. *Low incidence of acute urinary retention in the general male population: the Triumph Project*. Eur Urol 2005;47(4):494-498.

Vespa J, Medina L, Armstrong DM. *Demographic Turning Points for the United States: Population Projections for 2020 to 2060*. US Department of Commerce, United States Census Bureau. Issued March 2018. Revised February 2020

Wadie BS, Ibrahim E-HI, de la Rosette JJ, Gomha M, Ghoneim M. *The relationship of the International Prostate Symptom Score and objective parameters for diagnosing bladder outlet obstruction. Part I: when statistics fail*. J Urol 2001;165:32-34.

Wagle N, Campbell C, Di Capua P, Kocher B. *A clinical pathway to well-being: putting patient priorities at the center of care*. Am J Accountable Care 2023;11(3):37-40.

Wasson JH, Reda DJ, Bruskewitz RC, Elinson J, Keller AM, Henderson WG. *A comparison of transurethral surgery with watchful waiting for moderate symptoms of benign prostatic hyperplasia*. N Engl J Med 1995;332:75-79.

Wei JT, Calhoun E, Jacobsen SJ. *Urologic diseases in America project: benign prostatic hyperplasia*. J Urol 2005;173:1256-1261.

Wein A. *Symptom-based diagnosis of overactive bladder: an overview*. CUAJ 2011;5(suppl 2).

Whitcomb EL, Nager CW. *Urodynamics: when is testing clinically useful?* The Female Patient 2009;34:43-48.

Wikipedia. *Definition of anamnesis, medical history, medical case*. Available at: https://en.wikipedia.org/wiki/Medical_history

Williams CM. *Using medications appropriately in older adults*. Am Fam Phys 2002;66(10):1917-1924.

Woodburne RT. *Structure and function of the urinary bladder*. J Urol 1960;84(1):79-85.

Wymer KM, Narang G, Slade A, Sharma V, Thao V, Borah BJ, et al. *Evaluation of the cost-effectiveness of surgical treatment options for benign prostatic hyperplasia*. Urology 2023;171:96-102.

Xiong Y, Zhang Y, Li X, Qin F, Yuan J. *The prevalence and associated factors of lower urinary tract symptoms suggestive of benign prostatic hyperplasia in aging males*. Aging Male 2020;23:1432-1439.

Yoosuf BT, Panda AK, Favas M, Bharti SK, Devana SK, Bansal D. *Comparative efficacy and safety of alpha-blockers as monotherapy for benign prostatic hyperplasia: a systematic review and network meta-analysis*. Sci Rep 2024;14:11116.

Young MJ, Elmussareh M, Morrison T, Wilson JR. *The changing practice of transurethral resection of the prostate*. Ann R Coll Surg Engl 2018;100:326-329.

Zderic SA, Wein A, Rohrman D, Gong CL, Nigro D, Haugaard N, et al. *Mechanisms of bladder smooth-muscle hypertrophy and decompensation: lessons from normal development and the response to outlet obstruction*. World J Urol 1998;16:350-358.

Made in the USA
Las Vegas, NV
07 May 2025

9b7cfe2d-d2e8-45d0-9b73-b1d87c5fc27aR01